Scientifically Guaranteed Male Multiple Orgasms and Ultimate Sex

Restart Natural Penis Enlargement, Eliminate Forever Premature Ejaculation, Erectile Dysfunction, Impotence and Enjoy Daily Orgasms

by

Alan Ritz

Outskirts Press, Inc.
Denver, Colorado

Disclaimer

The information provided in this publication is for educational and informational purposes only and does not serve as a replacement to care and medical advice provided by your own personal health care team or physician. The author does not render or provide medical advice, and no individual should make any medical decisions or change their health behavior based on information provided here. Readers are encouraged to confirm the information contained herein with other sources. Readers should review the information in this publication carefully with their professional health care provider. Reliance on any information provided by the author is solely at your own risk.

The author does not recommend or endorse any specific products, medication, procedures, opinions, or other information that may be presented in the book. The author does not control information, advertisements, content, and articles provided by discussed third-party information suppliers. The author accepts no responsibility for materials contained in the book that you may find offensive. You are solely responsible for using the material contained in the authored publications in compliance with the laws of your country of residence, and your personal conscience. The author will not be liable for any direct, indirect, consequential, special, exemplary, or other damages arising from the use of information contained in this or other publications.

The author represents and warrants that s/he either owns or has the legal right to publish all material in this book. If you believe this to be incorrect, contact the publisher through its website at www.outskirtspress.com.

Scientifically Guaranteed Male Multiple Orgasms & Ultimate Sex
Restart natural penis enlargement, Eliminate forever premature ejaculation, erectile dysfunction, impotence and Enjoy daily orgasms
All Rights Reserved Copyright © 2005 Alan Ritz

Outskirts Press
http://www.outskirtspress.com

ISBN-10: 1-59800-168-X
ISBN-13: 978-1-59800-168-6

Library of Congress Control Number: 2005934572

Outskirts Press and the "OP" logo are trademarks belonging to Outskirts Press, Inc.
Printed in the United States of America

Table of Contents

Introduction

Achieve and enjoy the **ultimate** sexual performance, abilities and pleasure a man can experience every day with or without a partner. This requires only learning the following **100% exclusive knowledge** plus taking a multi-vitamin/mineral formula. I am a scientist who sticks to exact numbers, verifiable scientific data, proven methods and guaranteed results. This is exactly what you are going to find in this book. At the end of it I have included **7 pages** with the used references from **leading** medical, urological and research journals as well as clinical studies from the USA, UK, Germany and Japan. This strengthens the **guarantee** for 100% reliability of the provided in some cases **scientific breakthrough** information.

Successful and dramatic improvement of the current parameters of your male sexual system, abilities and pleasure will need **72 hours**. It occurs easily, precisely and more than anything else **safely**. Probably you have already heard of 2 FDA prosecuted sex pills manufacturers and the horror stories from the penis enlargement exercises, pumps and weights, which cause **erectile dysfunction** (impotence) and **premature ejaculation**. I have covered in A-Z details these 2 common problems and have explained why they occur. This is immediately followed by **100% scientific, free/cheap and permanent solutions**. To prove that I am <u>loyal only to you</u> and care entirely for your best interest, you will **not** find even one mentioning of any brand supplements, exercises, products, etc. I have not revealed even the brand of my preferred multi-vitamin/mineral formula because my goal is to fully educate you and then step back. **You** will know perfectly well what is the very best for your particular condition, needs and goals.

During my work with **The VIP Muscle®**, which is the male's multi orgasms generator, I found that a **side effect** is a **natural penis enlargement**. If you are endowed, I share how you can limit it as much as possible. If you consider it beneficial, there are detailed steps and advice on how to stimulate it for permanently adding approximately 1-1.5 inches. Note that this is the **natural restarted growth from your teen years**. It will keep on gradually increasing the length and width of your penis. That's why I strongly recommend to everyone who reaches **7 inches** (18 centimeters) to strictly limit this growth.

Everything in the book is clear, simple and to the point. I have taken as a **benchmark** the biochemical, hormonal and overall condition of a 20 years old male body. My objective is to show you how exactly to come back to that level and maintain it for the rest of your life. At that period your sexual system and whole body are in top condition. Plus, there are still excellent conditions for further natural penis enlargement. Once you reverse your biochemistry to this point, you can start enjoying **10+ orgasms** a day due to The VIP Muscle. Now let's start with the **3 factors** which determine your penis size and the ultimate peak in your sexual performance, health and abilities.

3 Factors Determine Your Penis Size and Ultimate Sexual Performance

There are 3 main factors, which determine the current size of your penis and the ultimate pleasure from its stimulation:

1. the concentration of **DHT** (de-hydro-testosterone) in your local penile tissues
2. the amount of the neurotransmitter **Acetylcholine** and erectile neurotransmitter **NO** (Nitric Oxide) in your genitals
3. the available blood volume and the output of your cardiovascular system

The Role of the Neurotransmitter Dopamine and Your Liver for the Production of DHT

The neurotransmitter **Dopamine** in your brain plays an essential role in the production of sufficient amounts of **testosterone**. This sex hormone is produced by your testicular and adrenal glands. Without enough Dopamine, the whole testosterone-producing chain in your body **cannot be unlocked**. These 2 glands produce pro-hormone

substances such as **DHEA** (de-hydro-epiandrosterone) and **cholesterol.** They have to be converted through several stages into **testosterone** and its final, super-potent form **DHT** (de-hydro-testosterone). The role of your **liver** is to provide the **enzymes,** which are necessary for these conversions. They also take part in the production of the crucial for the proper functioning of your nervous and sexual system neurotransmitters: **Acetylcholine, Serotonin** and **Dopamine**.

The Important Preventive Role of the Neurotransmitter Serotonin for Premature Ejaculation

The major role, which the neurotransmitter **Serotonin** plays, is to control and prevent excessive conversion of **Dopamine** (norepinephrine) into **Adrenaline** (epinephrine). Probably you know it as the "Stress hormone", because it unlocks the body for the "Fight or Flight" state. When it comes to sexuality, this results in premature ejaculation or erection withdrawal. That's why it is essential to maintain the conversion of Dopamine into Adrenaline at a minimum for optimum ejaculation control and prolonged sex. You can easily achieve this with the help of **Serotonin**. Sufficient amounts of it give your pituitary, testicular and adrenal glands the necessary time to produce a burst of **DHEA**. Then, the enzymes from your liver will convert it into testosterone and its final form **DHT**. Finally, it will power up your erection (and penis enlargement) from **the inside.**

What are the 2 Serious Health Problems Caused by DHT

For several years clinical studies have pointed out DHT as the cause for **prostate enlargement** and **male pattern baldness**. That's why it is a must to prevent its binding to the corresponding receptors in your prostate and scalp as well as to regularly detoxify your body from it. The secret for this is the **Dopamine** controlled production of Adrenaline.

The unique penile sponges contain numerous DHT receptors. This allows them to safely trap large amounts of it. This is one of the major requirements for 100% natural penis enlargement. To sum up, at the places where this super potent form of testosterone binds, the result is **enlargement**. Therefore, you may encourage and pursue it in your penile tissues but avoid it at your **prostate and scalp**.

What are the Natural Solutions to the DHT's Side Effects- Prostate Enlargement and Male Pattern Baldness

Clinical tests show that substances called **isoflavones** and several antioxidants successfully prevent DHT from binding in the receptors around your prostate and scalp. Furthermore, they can detoxify it from your body. You can supply the following **4** crucial for preventing or reversing prostate enlargement and male pattern baldness substances:

1. **isoflavones** from Saw Palmetto and Soy
2. **bioflavonoids** from Citrus fruits
3. **polyphenols** from Grape's seeds and peel
4. **lycopene** from Tomatoes

They are part of every advanced multi-vitamin/mineral formula. As a general rule, make sure that you also eat a lot of nuts, seeds, vegetables and fruits. They contain many unique antioxidants and bioactive substances, which will successfully protect and detoxify your body.

The 4 Requirements for Successful Restarted Penis Enlargement and Ultimate Sexual Performance

Your whole body, which means **all** your systems, glands and organs, must be super-charged and very potent. This has to happen **before** you can enlarge your penis and/or prepare your sexual system for an ultimate, multi-orgasmic performance **24/7/365**. Let's see how exactly to "enlarge" each of your systems and organs. For your convenience I have presented the details in the form of requirement - problems - explanations - solutions.

Requirement N1- Spontaneous Erection

You have to reach a **spontaneous erection** with nothing more than a gentle warming massage of your overall genital area **without** even touching your penis.

Problem: You need direct stimulation of your penis to get an erection.

Explanation: The Parasympathetic nervous endings in your penis lack enough amount of the neurotransmitter **acetylcholine**. As a result, the production of the **erectile neurotransmitter NO** (Nitric oxide), which is the precursor of the **erectile dilator cGMP** (cyclic Guanosine Monophosphate), **cannot** be unlocked. cGMP is responsible for exciting the arteries in the penile sponges to fill and fully expand millions of tiny interconnected blood chambers in your penis. As the penile shaft becomes larger, the veins in it are squeezed for an almost one way blood flow. The start of NO and cGMP production requires the neurotransmitter **acetylcholine**. Without it the result is **erectile dysfunction (impotence)**!

Solution: Find out below which of the 2 substances powering your erection causes this problem:

1. Acetylcholine
2. NO/cGMP

Explanation of the Mechanism Behind Your Erections

The whole process behind the erection starts with the presence of **acetylcholine** in the parasympathetic nerves in your genitals and penis. That's why, if you have a **pain** in its base or body even if you press it slightly, this is a reliable indicator for a **damage** of these nerves. They rely heavily on Acetylcholine to function properly. The second indicator for the available amount of this neurotransmitter is the **angle of your erection**. If it is horizontal or even downward, then surely you are **severely deficient of Acetylcholine**.

The Only Natural Solution within 2-3 Days to Erectile Dysfunction (Impotence) caused by Insufficient Acetylcholine

In each of the two cases mentioned above, all you have to do is simply provide your body with supplements, which act as **choline** donors. You can find them in high quality multi-vitamin/mineral formulas and in mood or memory enhancing supplements. One of the most common donor is **phosphatidylcholine**, which comprises 20-30% of **Lecithin**. The other two are **choline chloride** and **choline bitartrate**. Both of them are "safe" according to the US Food and Drug Administration (for reference you can go online at www.cfsan.fda.gov/~lrd/fcf182.html)

A word of caution. On this FDA list you can find substances, which are **not** completely harmless. A typical example is caffeine. Even choline bitartrate in large doses may cause increased acidity in your stomach or diarrhea. As a supplement, it is usually offered as a powder. That's why if you start using it, take the daily dose into 2-3 smaller doses mixed with juice or water after meals.

For fastest conversion of choline to Acetylcholine, **Pantothenic acid,** also known as **Vitamin B5,** is needed, as well as a little bit of Vitamin C. Since choline is easily oxidized, mix it with (fresh) fruit juices, which are rich in antioxidant nutrients. If it is not possible, after you mix it, drink it **immediately** to reduce the exposure to Oxygen. Regardless of the initial substance supplying the choline, your body will produce from it the neurotransmitter Acetylcholine. Thus, it will nurture and power your whole Parasympathetic nervous system.

According to FDA the AI (Adequate Intake) of choline is **550 mg/day** for men. The "Tolerable Upper Intake Level" (UL) for adults is **3.5 g/day**. The critical adverse effect from higher intake is hypotension (low blood pressure), with "sweating, diarrhea and fishy body odor". For more information http://www.cfsan.fda.gov/~dms/flcholin.html (to insert the specific character "~" at the web address press Shift and the button **above** "Tab" on the keyboard)

You should know as much as possible about such substances before taking them. The point is to maximize the benefits from a substance and minimize any possible adverse effects. **Your health is mainly in your hands.** FDA and other similar agencies do their best to provide reliable health-related information. However, you and your body are unique. That's why if something is good for the majority of people this does **not** mean that it will be good for you as well.

My best piece of advice is to keep learning and educating yourself. Once you understand how exactly your body works, the solution to certain serious and common problems such as erectile dysfunction, can be as simple as changing your current multi-vitamin formula with a choline containing one!

Nowadays, I witness the rise of a very serious problem. Urologists, sex pills producers, men's magazines, etc. have **no** financial interest to write and really help men to **permanently solve** such type of problems. The reason is that they easily become chronic. Then you have to buy time and again expensive Viagra or sex pills, which practically do **not** provide a permanent solution.

What to do in the other case: Erectile Dysfunction caused by Insufficient Production of NO/cGMP

The parasympathetic nerves can excite the arteries to start filling the blood chambers in your penis. As a result it becomes bigger but does **not** rise upward. In this case the problem is due to **insufficient production** of **NO** and **cGMP**. I will give you some important preliminary information to make it easier to understand the simple solution.

From HGH (Human Growth Hormone) to Erectile Dilator cGMP– Explanation of the Conversions

The growth of every organ and system, including your penis, is directly related to the daily released amount of HGH (Human Growth Hormone) from the pituitary/thyroid glands in your body. After 21, when the production of **HGH** and **Testosterone/DHT** reaches the peak in a man's life, their quantity gradually starts to decrease.

Clinical studies have proved that the **amino acid L-Arginine** has the ability to act as a moderate HGH releaser. As a result, now you can find it in most of the anti-aging, anti-obesity and bodybuilding formulas. From infancy till adulthood, the growth of muscle and penile tissues is directly related to the amounts of **HGH** and **DHT** in your body.

The **pituitary gland** in your brain has a direct impact on your testicular and adrenal functions. That's why a decrease in its functions leads to decrease in the production of testosterone and DHT. As a result, men's interest towards sex and their ability for it decline with the years.

The Role of HGH and the Amino Acid L-Arginine in the NO Production

The production of **NO** (Nitric Oxide) requires abundance of Nitrogen. It is supplied by the available in the blood HGH and L-Arginine in the penile and genital tissues. It reacts with the Oxygen from your blood to form the **erectile neurotransmitter NO**. Once there is enough amount of it, in the penile arteries starts the synthesis of **cGMP** (cyclic Guanosine Monophosphate). This is the erectile dilator and is **crucial** for having and holding an upward erection.

As you can see, everything narrows down to whether you have enough cGMP in your penile tissues or not, unless there is a deficiency of Acetylcholine to start the whole process.

The Natural Solution within 2-3 Days to Erectile Dysfunction caused by Insufficient NO/cGMP

The solution is again simple. You need abundance of the amino acid **L-Arginine** in your blood. There are two ways to supply it. The first one is through the **amino acid L-Ornithine**, which is the precursor, and your body will make L-Arginine from it. The other way is to include in your diet a supplement containing L-Arginine. Both amino acids have the additional benefit of boosting the release of human growth hormone. For a complete list of the health benefits of L-Arginine, take a look at The Directory of Vital Substances later on in the book.

Phosphorus is an important part of the chemical formula of cGMP. That's why your multi-vitamin/mineral formula should provide at least 100% of the **US RDA** (Recommended Daily Allowance). Another possible problem is that you may have sufficient amount of Nitrogen donating (HGH, L-Arginine, L-Ornithine), but your blood may not provide sufficient amount of **Oxygen** for the production of NO. To avoid such deficiency, make sure that there is a lot of fresh air in the room you use for sexual activities. Furthermore, breathe deeply from the beginning till the end to maximize the available Oxygen in your blood.

Heavy smokers are guaranteed to suffer from Oxygen deficiency due to the **400 toxic elements** from the cigarette smoke, which clog their lungs and saturate their blood. This is the mechanism through which cigarettes cause in the long term impotence.

Sometimes related is **Iron deficiency** because red blood cells need it to transport the Oxygen. The solution is to take **50-100%** of the US RDA. This mineral deserves special attention. The RDA dose is **18 mg**. If you use several supplements, the overall amount of iron you take in a single day must be <u>less than 45 mg</u>. This is FDA's upper tolerable intake. However, men do **not** need a lot of supplemental iron because they get enough from food.

To sum up, you need to supplement Nitrogen donating (L-Ornithine, L-Arginine or boost HGH), and the minerals Phosphorous and Iron. The only missing factor is clean, fresh air rich in Oxygen in the room whenever you have sexual activity. This combination permanently eliminates erectile dysfunction (impotence) due to NO/cGMP deficiency. After that, a **protein-rich diet**, which provides all amino acids, and an **advanced** multi vitamin/mineral formula are enough to secure an upright erection every time.

Requirement N2- Bursts of Testosterone Converted to DHT

The second requirement for a restarted natural penis enlargement and ultimate sexual performance is bursts of testosterone, converted into DHT. This ensures the **rock hardness** of your penis throughout the entire sexual activity.
Problem: Your pituitary, testicular and adrenal glands **cannot** produce enough pro-hormones such as DHEA

from cholesterol or your liver **cannot** supply the necessary enzymes for their conversion into DHT.

Explanation 1: The neurotransmitter **Dopamine**, which is the key to unlocking this testosterone-producing chain, is **deficient** in your body. There can be 2 reasons for that. Your answer to the following 2 questions will immediately reveal the source of the problem.

- Do you often feel anxiety, nervousness, mood swings and even panic attacks without having a logical and obvious reason for that? If your answer is positive, the problem is most probably due to **serious deficiency of Serotonin.** Its role is to preserve the conversion of Dopamine into the stress hormone **Adrenalin,** which causes problems with anxiety, tension, sleeplessness, moodiness and anti-social behaviour.

Solution: It is only one- you need a lot of **Serotonin** to reduce the production of Adrenalin from Dopamine. Your body produces it from the precursor **5-HTP** (5-hydro-tryptophan), which is made from the essential **amino acid tryptophan**. Once the deficiency is gone, you will feel much calmer and relaxed. At a sexual level your problems with premature ejaculation will also fade away and you will **endure much longer**.

Personally, I use a pharmaceutical grade 5-HTP supplement <u>only</u> when I have a very stressful occasion such as negotiations, presentation in front of many people or when my girlfriend wants more than 1-hour sex. In this third case I also add 100-200 mg **GABA** (Gamma-Amino-Butyric-Acid) dissolved in juice or water, preferably on an empty stomach. If the case is urgent, I dissolve it in my mouth for faster assimilation. The taste is almost neutral. Take it on an empty stomach or wait 1 hour after meal. It should **not** be taken with milk, meat or other protein-rich foods as well as with hot fluids.

GABA increases the selective responsiveness of the nerves towards external stimuli. In sexual terms, it **slows down** the unlocking of the ejaculation process and helps men to **be in control much longer.** The partially decreased activity of the neurotransmitters (and level of pleasure) is compensated by the length of the sex.

Please, **do not** use great doses of supplemental GABA (more than 350 mg) because instead of 1-2 hours' sex, you may fall asleep. Once again the **main substance** against premature ejaculation is **Serotonin**. Combine it with Acetylcholine and a little bit of GABA when you need extra enduring power.

Your body can use 5-HTP only for the production of **Serotonin** with the help of **Vitamins B-2** (Riboflavin), **B-3** (Niacin) and **especially B-6** (Pyridoxine), which maximize and speed up its production. FDA warns that very high doses of **Niacin and B-6** lead to serious damages of different parts of the body. That's why be cautious with them.

Furthermore, there are cases of people who have used manufactured **tryptophan** and have developed EMS- a potentially fatal disorder of the connective tissue and blood. It seems that 5-HTP supplements are preferable, although FDA does **not** consider them completely safe because of EMS. That's why my advice as usual is to be careful. If you have Serotonin/Dopamine deficiency then you need to take pharmaceutical grade 5-HTP at least for several days. Once the problem is gone, **stop** taking it.

If you use protein-rich source of amino acids such as **whey protein** then everything is all right. The L-tryptophan and L-phenylalanine, which naturally occur in it, are protein-bind and are considered **safe**.

- Do you feel calm, relaxed and in good ejaculation control? If your answer is positive, the reason for the sluggish production of testosterone in your body is probably due to **deficiency of Dopamine**.

Solution: This issue is also very easy to solve by supplying in your diet one of Dopamine's precursor - the **amino acid L-tyrosine**. If you have high blood pressure, consult your physician before taking **L-Tyrosine**. The reason is that Dopamine and Adrenalin, which are produced from them, can cause smooth muscular and arterial contractions, which may raise the blood pressure. You have probably noticed that when you are under stress your muscles become quite stiff.

Furthermore, if you suffer from insomnia, avoid taking this amino acid before going to bed because of its stimulating effect. Please, refer to the Directory of Vital Substances for in-depth information and **Frequently Asked Questions** regarding all substances I mention throughout the book.

Explanation 2: If the levels of Serotonin and Dopamine in your body are normal, the problem is most probably caused by a sluggish work of your **liver**. With regard to your sexual system, its main function is to supply the enzyme **5-alpha-reductaze**, which makes the conversion of testosterone into DHT. That's why if you have an upward erection (Acetylcholine), your penis fills with blood and becomes bigger (NO/cGMP) though it remains **soft,** the problem is exactly **insufficient DHT conversion**. It makes an erected penis **hard** and **hot**.

Solution: Your liver, which is responsible for this, is **not** driven well by your Parasympathetic nervous system. The reason for this is **deficiency of Acetylcholine.** The solution is to provide your body with at least 550 mg/

day choline from a multi-vitamin/mineral formula and/or single-substance supplement.

Requirement N3- High Blood Volume and Reliable Cardiovascular Support

You need **abundance of blood** and reliable cardiovascular support of your erection.

Problem: You are often pale, your hands and feet are regularly cold. You unintentionally keep yourself thirsty, your heart has become **lazy** from sedentary lifestyle or your blood pressure is too high or low. aggravate

Explanation 1: You are **severely blood deficient** and this can easily spoil any efforts for the improvement of your sexual abilities and overall health. At the same time, of all the discussed problems this is **the easiest** to solve. The reason is that all of these neurotransmitters, hormones and enzymes have to reach your penis/genital area. The only way is through your blood. What happens when your body needs water but you do not provide it? It takes out from the first internal source- your **blood**, which consists of about **80% water**.

Solution: Men with western type of lifestyle or mindset may find it difficult to drink enough to satisfy the need for water of their bodies. However, if you are really serious about achieving and after that maintaining top sexual condition, you need **minimum 2.5 liters/85 fl. oz daily**. The temporary effect on your sexuality from $50 sex or weight loss pills can be similar but the difference in price, duration of intake and naturalness of both ways is **huge**.

Requirement N4- Excellent Ejaculation Control

You need excellent ejaculation control of **minimum 30 minutes.** Furthermore, it is a must during an intercourse or masturbation to come very close to ejaculation at least **3-4 times** but remain in control, calm down a little bit and continue again. Why is this so important? Probably you have noticed that at the time of ejaculation the length and gird of your penis is expanded to **maximum**.

You should prepare your body by loading it with all the necessary substances to successfully keep a hard, hot and upright erection for 30-60 minutes. Then 3-5 times per sex or masturbation for 1-2 minutes, come close to ejaculation. Exactly at this time your fully loaded penis with rich in DHT blood will naturally and gradually **enlarge.** The two reasons are the great blood pressure inside it and the building of new DHT receptors in the shaft.

In this way you create the perfect environment for growth by having great amount of blood in the penis, which is very rich of Oxygen, 5-alpha-reductaze for local DHT conversion, NO/cGMP and amino acids, which are the building blocks for new receptors.
Problem: You have little or no control over your ejaculations- **premature ejaculation**.
Explanation: Your whole body is set for "Fight or Flight" state due to a lot of Adrenaline in your body. The effect on your nervous system is unreasonable anxiety, depression or aggression and mood swings. At the level of your sexual system it results in **premature ejaculation** (Fight) or **erection dysfunction** (Flight).
Solution: The ultimate goal is to dramatically reduce the quantity of Adrenaline in your body. As you already know the control is exerted by **Serotonin/Dopamine.**

Summary of the Minimum Requirements

To sum up, you need at the **minimum:**

- a nervous system fully loaded with **Acetylcholine, Serotonin** and **Dopamine**, which can successfully start and coordinate all biochemical and physiological processes in your body
- penis, fully loaded with blood rich in **Oxygen, 5-alpha-reductaze** enzyme for local **DHT** conversion, **NO, cGMP** and **amino acids** for hard, erection and ejaculation control.
- a powerful cardiovascular system, which has available abundance of blood to pump in your penis and genitals.
- properly functioning pituitary, testicular and adrenal glands and liver, which are perfectly driven by **Acetylcholine** and your Parasympathetic nervous system.

How to Fight Deficiencies of the Top 3 Substances and Obesity

Probably you have already wondered about the factors, which contribute to the deficiency of the major biosubstances I refer to all the time. After all, is it necessary to take some particular supplement all your life? Here are the answers for each of the **Top 3 substances**.

Acetylcholine

This deficiency is one of the most widely spread. At the same time it is **very cheap and easy** to end it with a choline-containing multi-vitamin/mineral formula and/ or single-substance supplement. Since this is the neurotransmitter of the Parasympathetic Nervous System, you need plenty of it every day to ensure its perfect functioning for:

- keeping you calm
- feeling full of energy
- having a clear mind
- driving properly your liver and metabolism
- starting the production of NO/cGMP for upright erection

A problem in any of these areas shows <u>serious deficiency</u> of Acetylcholine.

Stress, obesity and regular sexual activity (with or without a partner) can easily deplete this substance. If you wonder why, try to guess how much Acetylcholine your body needs just to maintain your erection for 30 minutes. And if you are multi-orgasmic, those millions of pleasurable sensations (nervous signals) have to go up to your brain through the spinal cord (parasympathetic nervous system). This requires **heavy doses** of this neurotransmitter. Within the nervous system, its role is to enable the communication between the neurons (nerves).

Let me give you an example with an Internet connection. If you have a computer, it is connected with your Internet Provider with a cable. When you plug it, you can immediately see the speed and quality of the transmitted information. The same is true for your parasympathetic nerves at your penis. They are connected with the spinal cord (parasympathetic nervous system) at the tailbone area and through it with the brain and the **center of pleasure** in it.

If there is deficiency of Acetylcholine, the communication (pleasure signals and sensations) between the genital nerves and the brain is **scrambled** and you are **not** actually feeling great pleasure (receiving many signals in the pleasure center) from sexual stimulation. Otherwise, it is just like a broadband connection because **100%** of the nervous signals instantly reach the brain with perfect quality! If you receive one and the same sexual stimulation with and without Acetylcholine deficiency I guarantee you that the difference in your feelings/pleasure will be **HUGE!**

Since the Parasympathetic Nervous System directly or indirectly manages **everything in the body,** proper amounts of choline are vital! FDA has already established this substance as **essential**. They have estimated that the daily need of choline for males between 9-13 years is **375 mg/day**. For men above 14 years it is **550 mg/day**.

I take the best multi vitamin/mineral formula, but even it does **not** provide more than 250 mg/day from it. That's why I take daily additional b **0.8-1 g** from a Lecithin, Vitamin B5 and BHA (beta-hydroxy-acid) supplement. There are choline-providing formulas, which contain "**Guarana**". This is a South American herb **2.5 times** richer of caffeine than coffee. If you see a supplement containing it I recommend that you skip it. You can find the complete information on this topic in the Directory of Vital Substances under **Caffeine**.

How can you know the precise amount of choline you need per day? This is one of the Top 3 substances, which have direct and indirect impact on every system and organ in your body. I use a simple criterion to determine whether a male body is in top condition. It is **spontaneous erections,** like the ones you had in your teens. I want to underline that your current age does **not** matter. You can still have them at **70+** as well as at 30!

Having spontaneous erections should be your **first goal**. Once you achieve it, the next one is to maintain your body in top condition and enjoy your erections. It is as simple as that. This book will assist you to achieve these 2 goals at a **minimal cost**, **naturally** and **effortlessly**. Acetylcholine is one of the key substances for achieving both targets.

Serotonin

From my observations I can say that nowadays the most sexually active males- teenagers and young adults are

severely deficient of Serotonin. This is also the main reason why it is so common to hear parents complaining from groundlessly depressed or aggressive teenager. This is all due to the fact that the significant amount of **Serotonin** released in the bloodstream immediately after ejaculation, converts to **Melatonin**.

Exactly during the first years of the puberty guys start ejaculating <u>too often</u> without taking **enough L-tryptophan** from their food. Another very common reason is the so called drug **Ecstasy**. Both factors automatically lead to <u>severe depletion</u> of Serotonin. Without it uncontrolled conversion of Dopamine into Adrenalin takes place 24 hours a day. This greatly fuels the "Fight or Flight" behaviour. The Serotonin-dependent **Dopamine** unlocks the whole testosterone-producing chain, which is of **fundamental importance** for every man. For better understanding here is Serotonin's whole chain of conversions: L-tryptophan (amino acid) – 5-HTP (5-hydro-tryptophan) - Serotonin – Melatonin.

In the evenings, the levels of Melatonin in the body naturally go up and cause the need for sleep. This is the reason why men often fall asleep after they have ejaculated. This is due to their biochemistry.

If you have deficiency of Serotonin, taking pharmaceutical grade 5-HTP will eliminate it within few days. However, there is something very simple, which you can do to prevent it from occurring again- **control your ejaculation frequency!** There is simply no other way! If you are under 19, you can safely ejaculate <u>up to 3 times </u>a week. If you are 20-35, you can safely ejaculate **2 times** a week. However, for both age groups there <u>must</u> be at least 1 day between 2 ejaculations!

<u>Never ejaculate more than 1 time per day!</u> Breaking this rule guarantees you **depletion** of your testicles,

Prostaglandin E-1 (PGE-1) and Serotonin stores. As you will read later on, I strongly recommend that every man take on a daily basis at least 1-2 tablets or soup spoons of <u>whey protein</u>. It provides all amino acids, including **safe natural L-tryptophan**. However, your testicles and PGE-1 are the two areas which over-ejaculation depletes <u>completely</u>. That's why whey protein can **not** neutralize the overall negative effect of over-ejaculation.

Men between 36-45 can safely ejaculate **once a week**. For those who are 46-50, the appropriate frequency is **once in 2 weeks**. For those in the age range 51-59 it is **once a month**. If you are over 60, maintain active sexual activity <u>without ejaculating any more</u>.

The highest level of sexual pleasure for 99.99% of men comes from those <u>few seconds</u> during ejaculation. Once your body is prepared (fully loaded with all major sub-stances) start using the **VIP Muscle®** for multiple or-gasms. You will immediately notice a **HUGE** difference compared to your sexual experience so far. Due to the VIP Muscle which I will discuss in details later, you will enjoy <u>pure ecstasy</u> from **multi-orgasmic** sexual activ-ity (with or without a partner). Yes, this is **exactly** what this book will help you to achieve. Then the next goal is to maintain and enjoy this state **till the rest of your life.** Now let's continue with the third substance.

Mineral Water

I bet that you have expected to see another substance in this Top 3 list. Probably **Dopamine,** but your body can produce it from the proteins from your food. Furthermore, if the levels of **Serotonin** are normal, it is quite difficult to end up with such deficiency. Even if it happens, this will affect mainly your testosterone production, which will only result in softer erections and faster aging.

If you expected it to be the enzyme **5-alpha-reductaze,** I have an excellent example. Some of the pills against male pattern baldness **block** its production. In this way they prevent more DHT to reach your hair-rooting cells preventing additional hair loss. The cost for this, however, is **erectile dysfunction** because of insufficient conversion of testosterone into DHT. After all, the hardness of your erection depends on that. The result usually is a severe damage to your male confidence and sexual abilities but nothing more.

You may be surprised why mineral water shares the spotlight with Acetylcholine and Serotonin. To support my nominee, I want to note that you can live only **3 minutes** without Oxygen, **3 days** without water and **1 week** without food. That's why water is <u>twice as important as food</u> and is the **second most important** substance to keep you alive. Now you probably understand why deficiency of water is a life-threatening condition! Every man who is conscientious about his health carries a (big) bottle full of mineral water with low mineralization. Also, he makes sure that it is **empty** by the end of the day.

Ultimate Sexual Performance versus Obesity

All right, you can solve any sexual problems such as

- erectile dysfunction (impotence)
- premature ejaculation
- lack of libido
- regular fatigue
- Acetylcholine/PGE-1 dependent low back pain

However, if you have extra 50-200 lbs (25-100 kg), it will not matter a lot, right? Do you currently starve yourself, run on Treadmills, follow strict/radical diets or take expensive pills with the only purpose to lose weight? If your answer is positive, please **stop**. Most of them are **totally wrong** and are **very harmful** for your body.

Have you ever seen an obese wild animal? Surely not and you will **not** see one. Being in perfect condition year after year is essential by nature to stay alive and pass your genes. Animals know how to do achieve it, though the "smart" human beings often fail.

People believe that the more they sweat the more fat they burn. This is a far cry from the truth. Actually, it is exactly the opposite! **Intensive exercises** (for example running quickly) seriously decrease their chances to lose fat. Such myths only aggravate their problem. Obese men need a solution so badly, that they try almost everything, even if it is **bad** for their health.

Applying the information from this book will help men to start reducing their extra pounds. There are certain principles about **weight management**, which every person should know. For example, the more you push your body to the extreme, the **more obese** you will become. You may ask: "Is there also some simple, free/cheap and entirely scientific/natural solution to obesity?" **Definitely yes** and you can already point some of the key factors.

Take a pen and a sheet of paper and think about "the solution" to **USA's #1 problem- obesity**. According to official data, **61%** of the American people over 16 are obese! With the information so far, you have around **50%** of the necessary scientific knowledge to **solve** it. 95% of the authors of "diets" can only dream to know that much. However, they are busier trying to convince people that

<u>speculations</u>, such as blood groups, types of metabolism, timing, high protein low carbs, etc. have something to do with **easy, fast, cheap and permanent** weight loss without starvation.

I wonder why there are still no diets for the different star signs. Probably because I am Leo I would have eaten some fancy "high protein low carbs" diet. All popular diets would be funny and interesting to read if there weren't **15 million morbidly obese people only in the USA!** The greater problem is that their only option is surgery, which is not affordable for the average person. This is the reason why my next book will be "**Your Scientific Diet for Men**", followed by an equivalent for women. Here are the key points and goals, which I challenged myself to achieve:

weight-optimizing scientific anti-diet- it must exceed the highest expectations of a morbidly obese man, a skinny teenager and a top Hollywood celebrity, who wish to maintain his top condition

reliable as a Swiss watch- strictly based on Biochemistry and mathematical formulas, which will help you to predict precisely how much and how fast you will reduce or increase your weight. And once you become absolutely satisfied, how to maintain it easily for the rest of your life.

you are in total control- you can select among 3 pre-calculated plans: 71, 143 or 214 grams of burnt fat/day to achieve a corresponding target of **0.5, 1.0 or 1.5 kg fat lose/week**. Also, you can use the mathematical formulas to make your own plan such as 200 g/day-1.4 kg/week for your convenience

flexible- applicable even in the hectic work environment at the NY Stock Exchange

affordable- perfectly affordable for the average man

no suffering- proves with scientific data and references why starving, reducing carbohydrates or calories and sexual inactivity severely damage the male body and lead to obesity and related impotence

total- targets a dynamic balance between the physical, emotional, mental and spiritual level and maintain them in constant harmony

personalized- I believe that every single person is unique. That's why there are no "one-size-fits-all" approaches and lists with "good" and "bad" foods.

results-dominance- my objective was to write the most affordable and customized scientific anti-diet, which will permanently burn up to 3.3 lbs. of fat (1.5 kg) per week

balanced- values not only the macro nutrients- water, carbohydrates, proteins and fats, but also the micro ones (vitamins and minerals). Every radical diet, which restricts or excludes certain macro nutrients, runs counter to our genetic heritage and damages the body for little or no permanent results.

100% science-based- free of any hypothetical elements (speculations). It helps you not only to loose or gain weight, but also to maintain it after that. (Every time I see a diet claiming that it is based on science, I expect to see that a skinny guy can gain weight with it as well. Pure science always works in 2 ways just like the atomic power can be used for generation of electricity and mass destruction. If a "scientific" diet claims to achieve only weight loss then this proves that it is **not** really science-based).

strings-free- I am loyal only to you and your best interest. That's why you will also **not** find recommendation for any particular product or company. In this way, I will continue to expose useless, expensive and harmful products, foods and drinks.

educational- A-Z scientific explanation as to how exactly the male body works and what it needs to optimize its weight and maintain it constantly

focused- everything is clear, simple and to the point

advanced- it is built upon "Scientifically Guaranteed Male Multiple Orgasms and Ultimate Sex"

does not depend on fitness- it is great if you make exercises. However, a sedentary lifestyle will **not** hinder a weight reduction goal. In case that you want to increase your muscle mass, fitness is essential.

The major substances play a major role in your sexual abilities and performance. They also determine how fit, sexy and healthy you are, regardless of your biological age!

My observations over aging men made me want to take actions against becoming also a victim of obesity, baldness and impotence. I challenged myself to find the answer to the ultimate question: "How can a man look like 25-30 without plastic surgery and maintain the biochemistry levels from his youth till the rest of his life?"

I achieved my goal and this book contains everything I know for being in such top condition 24/7/365. I dedicated my next book **Your Scientific Diet®** to all the men and women who face the challenge to manage their weight.

Now let's continue with several advanced principles necessary for a man willing to restart the natural penis enlargement from his teens.

Advanced Principles for Restarting and Accelerating Natural Penis Enlargement

The first key substance, which can **dramatically** improve the common male sexual problems (impotence and premature ejaculation) as well as your performance and penis size, is **Acetylcholine**. You can supply the precursor of this **most important neurotransmitter** from **choline**-containing supplements. As you have seen so far, your whole body must be completely healthy and in a very good condition. Without this, any enlargement attempts will only damage or shrink your penis. The result is one of the top 3 male sexual problems- erectile dysfunction, premature ejaculation or deformations.

Just think for a moment. Did you use something (exercises, pills, pumps or extenders) from 9-16 to grow your penis to its current size? Surely not. It has grown naturally with 2-3 inches for around 10 years in your teens. That's why the normal growth rate is around 0.4-0.5 inches per year!

The Penis is Not a Muscle!

This anatomical fact explains why the whole idea for "exercises" or "penile fitness" is **fundamentally wrong** and leads only to devastating results. The internal structure of your penis consists of huge number of tiny blood vessels and chambers. There is no muscle or something, which you can **mechanically stretch.** You can only **break** the delicate spongy tissues and blood vessels as well as damage the parasympathetic nerves. The result from such masochistic activities is guaranteed decreased sensitivity, redness or even impotence.

Now do you realize that all those sites, which promise 3 inches in just few weeks, know nothing about the **real**, **natural** and most importantly **safe** approach to penis enlargement? You need the support of your nervous and cardiovascular system, glands and liver. Otherwise, starting any method, which applies force on the inflatable blood structures in the penis, will only result in their **temporary or permanent damage**.

Natural penis enlargement occurs automatically from maintaining/restarting the top biochemical condition from your puberty. This is all you have to do. The information provided in this book will help you to achieve exactly this. Also, you can use **The VIP Muscle**. For those who want to further encourage and speed up the enlargement, I have summarized the major steps below.

The F.A.S.T. System to Restart Your Penis Enlargement from Your Teens

-   focus on the neurotransmitters, pro-hormones, water and amino acids, which your body needs **in abun-**

dance to support any kind of "enlargement" and improvement.

- anticipate your body's needs. Find out from the book exactly which essential substances lack and supply them in your diet. In addition to the presented information above, read carefully the additional details from the Directory of Vital Substances given later on. As you have probably noticed, taking a **choline**-containing formula with **all** vitamins and minerals in safe quantities is a **must** for every man, carrying for his health and ultimate sexual performance.

- start doing regularly "**The VIP Massage**" for optimum blood circulation in your testicles, penis and genitals. Notice that what I have described below is strictly a **massage** and **not** "exercise" or masturbation.

The VIP Massage of the Genitals

The best time to do it is **after taking a shower**. Take your left testis with all of your fingers and start massaging its entire surface. After 1 minute take your right testis and do the same. In 1 minute go back to the left one. Follow this pattern for 5-6 minutes.

This is an excellent way to improve the blood circulation in your testicles and stimulate their production of **testosterone** and **sperm**. Avoid doing it for longer time, because your testicles have to stay <u>cool</u>. This is the main reason why it is bad to wear tight underwear. It keeps them close to your body, which heats them up. This affects their testosterone and sperm production.

Continue with the PC muscle just below your testicles. Massage slowly its right side and then its other side down to your anus. Massage clockwise with the tips of your fingers. Have in mind that built-up tension in this muscle often causes **premature ejaculation**. The reason is its direct connection with the **sympathetic nerves** in your genitals, which start and execute the ejaculation process.

Try to **avoid its contraction** as much as possible. Whenever you feel a need to urinate, do it as soon as possible. To hold it means to keep this muscle contracted **for hours**. Thus the accumulated tension may seriously interfere with your ejaculation control during sex. The **VIP Genital Massage** is an excellent and easy way to reduce the tension in this important muscle.

The next step is to massage the area around the base of your penis. Start from the right side by gently massaging it with the tips of your right fingers. Slowly move up to the middle and then move to the left side. After a while start using the tips of your left fingers to continue the massage from the left side.

The area at the base of the penis is **very important** because all arteries, veins and parasympathetic nerves connected to your penis come from here. That's why there must be **no blood congestions** or **scar tissues**. A reliable indicator for their presence is a curve at the base or the body of your penis. This problem is already difficult to fix. The solution **is possible** with the help of a little known substance in your body.

The Secret for a Perfectly Straight and Massive Penis- Prostaglandin E-1 (PGE-1)

Have you seen in your local drug store supplements called "**Evening Primrose Oil**" or "**Borage (Starflower)**

Oil"? Recently they have become popular, especially among women as a relief of post-menstrual syndrome and menstrual cramps. They also ease low back pain and **joint-related problems** such as rheumatoid arthritis. The effect on **skin elasticity** is also great. (A word of caution: epileptics should consult their doctor before taking supplements containing such oils.)

All these effects are due to **Gamma-Linolenic Acid (GLA)**. It is essential for the production of Prostaglandin E-1 in the body, which regulates several functions. Its N1 benefit for the men is an increase in the elasticity and stretching abilities of all nerves and blood vessels in your penile tissue. This is the last key factor for creating the <u>perfect environment</u> for the enlargement of your penis.

When the penile tissue is enriched with **all** vital substances, **new DHT receptors will form** and will expand your penis. At the same time, you <u>must</u> provide plenty of Prostaglandin E-1 to support this enlargement. Its role is to continuously increase the elasticity of the penile tissue and **suppress** the release of hardening collagen.

In your teens you had abundance of DHT and naturally high levels of Prostaglandin E-1. However, if you have been circumcised, this will restrict to some extend the maximum enlargement you can otherwise achieve. PGE-1 can slightly help the stretching of your remaining skin. In this way, you can go beyond the skin-fixed ultimate size.

Collagen is a substance, which is responsible for your skin thickness and relatively hard structure. With age the level of PGE-1 decreases faster than that of collagen. The result is hardening and wrinkling of the skin. Gradually the level of collagen also starts decreasing. This results in thinning of the skin, which becomes dry and wrinkled.

Some Gamma-Linolenic Acid donors such as Evening Primrose or Borage (Starflower) oil can slow this process down. Your body will convert it into Prostaglandin E-1, which will help to preserve the elasticity and youthful condition of your entire skin for a long time.

You can apply on your penis GLA rich oil during regular VIP Genital Massages. This will suppress the release of hardening collagen as a result from the restarted penis enlargement. Collagen is one of the major ways your body uses to stop your penis from becoming too big. Otherwise, at a rate of 0.4-0.5 inches/year imagine how long it can become if you live 80 years.

Here is the best plan for penile development. At 19, which is the end of your teens, it is best to have a **6 inch** penis. In the following years due to the vacuum effect of vaginal sex and, if necessary, by using GLA rich oil, you can further enlarge it up to **7 inches**. If you lose 2 inches until the age of 60, you will still have 5 inches, which is the average.

How to Limit Penis Enlargement

PGE-1-Collagen is the major way to limit penis enlargement when you do not want it any more. How can you do that? Simply **stop** applying oil rich in Gamma-Linolenic Acid on your penis as well as taking such orally usually in the form of soft gels. The second way is to switch to **collagen-boosting** cream or lotion. In this way, you will fix the size you have already achieved. However, have in mind that it will **not** stay like that until the end of your life.

The first reason for this is the destruction of collagen in your whole skin. That's why after you pass 30-35, it is very important to start using collagen-replenishing cream. It will maintain the necessary levels of this important substance in your skin. Use it on your face, neck, hands and penis.

The second reason for age-related shrinking of the penis is the so called **Andropause**. It is associated with a sharp decrease in the produced amount of testosterone in middle-aged men. Also, damaged/destroyed DHT receptors in your penis are **not** replaced and with the years, they become less and less. This combination automatically leads to shrinking. Starting from the age of 25, and especially in your 30s, **if you do nothing**, you are about to lose **1 inch** of the length of your penis. However, you are already perfectly prepared by this book to fight that natural process.

It will be a challenge if your starting size is already 7 inches, especially in your teens. In that case, you should **not** allow any further growth. How can you do that? Do **not** use GLA rich oil and limit the number of times you contract your VIP Muscle as much as possible. The reason is that it aggressively stimulates the chain Acetylcholine-NO-cGMP-maximum expansion of your penis. This is another reason why it is **better** to start with 5.5-6 inch penis. Then you can enjoy thousands of orgasms in the following years due to the VIP Muscle without worrying about the resulting enlargement.

The Official Average Size and When You Must Stop Enlarging Your Penis

Nowadays, men have a very distorted view of what is normal for a penile size. That's why it is important to know the official "average" in the world. Here are the results from a study published in Journal of Urology in

September, 1996. It concluded that the average flaccid penile length is **3 1/2 inches (8.8 cm.)**, while the average length in erection is **5 inches (12.8 cm.)**. The famous Kinsey Institute gives practically the same result.

"Size matters or does it?" this is the common question. For me it definitely matters and I am sure it is the same for you. Women on the other hand cannot give exact answer. Once a penis is inside, they cannot say precisely what its length is, which puts the stress on **how you use** your penis. Men from porn movies have penises above the average. After all, this is the main reason to be hired. However, because of softness, downward erection and inappropriate sex positions the pleasure they give is **minimal**.

Keep in mind that **average means normal**. In addition, it is better to have less than 7 inches before you start using the **VIP Muscle** for multiple orgasms. A rock hard, upright and long-lasting erection will drive any woman completely wild even if it is 5 inches long! I am sure that men who dream to have 8-10 inches believe that this will compensate some weakness in their abilities or performance.

Think about that and from biochemical point of view. Achieving such abnormal size requires **too much bioresources** such as neurotransmitters, hormones, enzymes, vasodilators and blood. Such great demand will put significant stress on your entire body on a daily basis. However, there is a second, even bigger problem. If the enlargement of your penis is done properly you will feel very virile. However, that long penis will cause **intense pain** to your partner!

The normal depth of the female vagina is **only 3-5 inches**! Imagine how easily a 9 inch penis, combined with powerful thrusts, may hurt the sensitive cervix or the bottom wall of the vagina. More important than enlarging your love tool 2-3 times more that she can handle, is to aim at having erection, which is:

- **maximum 7 inches**
- **rock hard**
- **up-right**
- **long-lasting**

That's it. Then your penis will continuously and powerfully stimulate the entire upper part of her vagina where are situated the 3 most sensitive points- the **Clitoris**, **G-spot** and near the bottom her **Cervix**. Even if you have a poor sexual education, having such erection will definitely win you the admiration of most of the women.

I doubt that there are many women in the world, who will agree to try a 10 inch penis. Starting from the ancient Chinese tradition, your **sexual health and education** (how you USE your penis) has always been considered more important than the size. Even if it is 4 inches you can perfectly trigger multiple orgasms in women. The reason is that you can still stimulate 2 of the 3 most sensitive points- her Clitoris and **G-spot,** which is situated 1-2 inches inside the vagina at the upper part. With a very long **but soft** or **flaccid** penis, it would be difficult even to get inside. That's why instead of dreaming about or going to extremes about your penis size, focus on the **Big Picture**.

Second Major Problem Associated with a Huge Penis- Male Pattern Baldness

Too long or massive penis will need the conversion of huge amount of testosterone into DHT every time you enjoy sex or masturbation. Without equally huge amounts of isoflavones, lycopene, polyphenols and antioxidants, you are almost bound to loose your hair in the near future. This is men's nightmare- **male pattern baldness**.

The perfect penis size for sex is between **5.5 - 7 inches**. If it is smaller, you may not be able to reach her third highly sensitive spot - the **Cervix** situated at the upper part of the vagina's bottom wall. On the contrary, if it is bigger you can press it too much, causing her pain and discomfort. In addition, it is very difficult to power a huge penis for a **rock hard and up-right erection**.

At the same time, this condition is necessary if you want to give maximum stimulation and multi-orgasms to your lady. The amount of Acetylcholine, which your body has to burn for only 15 minutes of sex or masturbation just to power it up, is **great**! This can leave your Parasympathetic nervous system with deficiency of its main neurotransmitter. The result will be decreased sensitivity and (serious) inability to perform its management functions in your whole body.

The **third victim** in this case will be your acetylcholine-driven liver. It will affect the production of 5-alpha-reductaze for smaller conversion of Testosterone into DHT, cause impotence and slow down **your entire metabolism**. If you already have problems with extra weight it will become even worse. Your liver is the General Manager of carbohydrates, fats, minerals and vitamins. If its performance is poor, this will reflect negatively how you feel and look.

Follow the Priority Table

The solution is to focus on the following **Priority Table.**

1. **hardness of your erection**
2. **up-right position**
3. **staying power and ejaculation control**
4. **circumference of your penis**
5. **length**

If, for example, the hardness decreases because of enlargement, you have to **stop it**. As you can see, the length is at the bottom and is the component, which will improve **only** after the previous 4 have improved or increased. At the same time it is the first, which will naturally decrease if you do nothing to counteract. Some men may disagree but the length is of least importance from biological and sexual point of view.

Learn from Hundreds of Horror Stories in Internet and Other Men's Mistakes

It is **full** across Internet with horror stories from penis enlargement exercises, pumps, weights, pills, extenders and surgery. The two most common complaints are **erectile dysfunction** and **deformation/curvature** of the penis either at the base or somewhere in the body. What specific damages occur as a result from using any of the **6 popular killers of penises?**

Killer N1- Penis Enlargement Weights

You attach to your flaccid, soft penis few pounds of weight and you can often hear a very clear sound- the sound, which announces **severe tearing** of your penile tissue, accompanied by <u>horrible pain</u>. Unfortunately, this single experience results in permanent impotence till the end of your life. This **fastest and most painful** method to become **completely impotent** starts from "only $49.95".

Killer N2- Penis Enlargement Pumps

You simply have to put your penis in it and start pumping. Men often go overboard thinking that the greater the vacuum, the faster and more significant gain in size. However, only the extent of the damage depends on the applied sucking power, because the length does not change. The vacuum breaks the walls of the blood vessels and even of the 2 main cylinders in the penis. This immediately leads to (**severe)** redness, swelling, (temporary) erectile dysfunction and a lot of **long-lasting pain**.

Killer N3 (Most Popular) - Penis Enlargement Exercises

I will quote a few sentences from several popular web sites. They start by describing in details Corpus Spongisum and Corpora Cavernosa. These are the two spongy cylinders in your penis. For men with limited sexual and anatomical education this introduction may look impressive and credible. But let's take a closer look of what follows.

They shamelessly confess that by making their exercises, you will **"break the walls of Corpus Cavernosa"** (the bigger cylinder, which is closer to your abdominals). For me this is more than enough to horrify me. However, it is interesting the way they try to twist it in order to trick men.

Probably you know that if you pump your muscles in a gym, there will be micro-tears in them. The body heals them internally within several days. As a result from the workouts your muscles become stronger and bigger. The site uses this fact by stating that "Your penis is not different from your muscles". Many men will probably see nothing suspicious in this and accept the penile fitness program.

They would expect for "just 49.95" to achieve "bigger and muscular penis", "excellent ejaculation control" and "doubled ejaculation volume". However, the result is **guaranteed** erectile dysfunction, decreased sensitivity and premature ejaculations. All "testimonials" on these sites are **fake** because the whole penile fitness concept is anatomically impossible! No man can apply external stretching force of any kind on his **inflatable penile tissue** without a **severe damage!** This is also clearly stated by **Alert: IA 7801** of the US Food and Drug Administration, which I will discuss in a while.

Killer N4- Penis Enlargement Surgery

What about this method, which starts from **$8,000**? Two studies made in 1994 and 1996 and published in the respected **Journal of Urology** reported significant complications from this type of surgery. Often there are **serious wound infections** and **penile deformity** such as lumpiness and asymmetry. The penile surgery is still unpredictable and controversial! At the same time the results are extremely poor. That's why it is considered **unacceptable** by both the urological and plastic surgery communities.

Let's see what the specific procedure and the consequences are. They cut exactly between the base of your penis and your abdominals. This **cuts off** the Parasympathetic nervous endings at your penis coming from the main Vagus nerve at your abdominals. The result is **insensitivity** towards sexual stimulation. Furthermore, it makes it **impossible** for these nerves to start local production of NO for erection and cGMP for holding it upright. All this means **permanent and irreversible impotence!** It looks crazy to me to pay $8,000 and loose your spontaneous upright erection **for ever.**

Besides, at the places of the cuts appear **scar tissues** because of the released collagen, which badly deform the shape of the penis. Taking and applying Evening Primrose/ Borage Oil and **Vitamin E** cannot fully neutralize this. In addition to erectile dysfunction and ugly deformations, this surgery often leads to **severe infections** because of the unpredictable and difficult to control complications. The waste products of bacteria metabolism in the wounds further damage the penile tissue.

Killer N5- Penis Enlargement Extenders

They are already advertised as an alternative to the methods mentioned above. I made a search at Google and was shocked by the prices- **up to $699 per gadget!** This type of device is incredibly simple. It has something like a "cock ring", which you have to place below the head and use the mechanism to keep your penis stretched for many hours. I was curious about the deceiving explanation of the method. Here is an exact quotation taken by a popular site: "When you gradually increase the longitudinal force on the shaft of the penis, the body's natural reaction to this force is multiplication of tissue cells and gradual expansion of the penile tissue. In other words, the penis gradually and naturally adds tissue for a larger and longer penis."

This explanation is provided by the two "medical doctors" behind the popular device and site. I am not a medical doctor and probably you are not as well. However, here is a small challenge. Let's find out **3 fundamentally wrong**

statements in it from **medical** and **anatomical** point of view.

Before this let's make a small experiment, which will prove how absurd is their statement. Take a clock, stop breathing and try to hold your breath for as long as you can. Any one will start breathing again within **2-3 minutes**. This is the maximum time the human body can survive without Oxygen. That's why it is the first and **most important** factor for staying alive. Although you wanted to hold your breath for a long time, you simply started breathing again.

You can't help it because of a specific center in your brain. It is irritated by increased concentration of Carbon Dioxide in your blood. You neither breathe out this gas nor supply fresh oxygen. That's why this center uses its direct connection with your respiratory system and orders it to start working again.

If someone ties around your neck a rope and hangs you, will you consider it beneficial for your health? Surely **not**. Due to the "orders" of the responsible center in the brain, you will struggle for breath for 2-3 minutes before you die from suffocation. Once you are dead, is it possible for any substance, manipulation or operation to bring you back to life? Except in the movies, the answer is **definitely not**.

With all this in mind, let's go back to the penis extender. You have to put its ring right below the head of your penis. Then the only way to stretch forward its body is to squeeze the head. Personally, I do not see any difference between hanging a person with a rope and hanging a penis with a tight "cock ring". Notice that once you set up the extender, you have to wear it under your clothes **day and night**.

Once the supply of Oxygen to your body is cut from a rope around your neck, how many minutes do you still have to live? Maximum 3. Regarding the need of Oxygen, "your penis is no different from your muscles". It is simply amazing and shocking the possibility to **pay $699 just to hang your penis!**

Let's go back to their "explanation". Did you already notice the 3 mistakes, which are shameful for "medical doctors"? "Reaction to this force is multiplication of tissue cells". First, the penis has a unique **spongy tissue**. It consists of millions of tiny interconnected blood **chambers, vessels, nerves** and **receptors** for DHT, touch, temperature and pain. Actually there are **no "tissue cells".**

Second, "**multiplication**" of any living organism such as a "cell" requires abundance of

- **oxygen**
- **amino acids**, which are the building blocks
- **minerals** for successful biochemical reactions

All these crucial factors are delivered by the blood flow, which these extenders seriously restrict.

Third, only the DHT receptors can multiply in your penis and you already know that this requires perfect environment and a lot of specific substances. Actually, a great part of the book so far has been dedicated on educating you how to achieve it. Only then can your body **build** new DHT receptors because they do **not** "multiply" as cells do. To state that the restriction of blood, oxygen and nutrients in the penile shaft will "multiply tissue cells" shows lack of knowledge about basic physiological principles and anatomy!

I think this is an excellent example about the kind of people who come up with many of the offers in the Internet. They will do their best to attract and deceive people. Unfortunately, those who believe them will **pay and suffer a lot**.

The Iron Back Up- FDA's Public Alert: IA 7801

I take the protection of your penis from such people and companies **extremely seriously**. That's why I want to impress on you that forceful methods for penis enlargement will not work for you. Now let's focus our attention on the **FDA's Public Alert: IA 7801**. (www.fda.gov/ora/ fiars/ora_import_ia7801.html)
The following is a quote, which provides its essence:

"The use of penis enlargers and erection maintaining rings may have **harmful effects**. They may aggravate existing medical conditions such as Peyronie's disease, Priapism, and urethral stricture. They may contuse or cause rupture of the subcutaneous blood vessels, which may produce hemorrhage and hematoma formation.

Prolonged use of the rings may cause gangrene of the penis. Basically, the labeling of these devices **falsely states or implies** they will treat impotence, prolong the erection and increase the dimensions of the penis. These devices generally fall into the following categories:

- mechanical stretching devices
- vacuum-operated devices
- constrictive rings
- supportive devices

INSTRUCTIONS: Unless exempted by Section 801.109, **automatically detain all devices in the categories mentioned above**". I think that the Food and Drug Administration is clear. As you can see, the potential complications are actually **worse** than I presented them here. If you develop gangrene, a surgeon will have to **cut off your penis!** At the same time, the source is the most trusted you could think of. At the time of this publication, the search engine Google gives 1,050,012 pages for the exact keyword phrase "penis enlargement". Can you image? There are already more than 1 million web pages competing to sell you expensive techniques and products, which will only lead to complications up to gangrene!

What are the Known and Hidden Dangers of Penis Enlargement Pills

The 5 penis killers discussed so far have one thing in common- they act externally. But you have probably heard about penis enlargement **pills**. Do they really work and do their producers hide the whole truth about their ingredients? As you will see, the situation is **not** much better than that with the other products and techniques. Now let's focus on a FDA's Warning provided at: www. fda.gov/bbs/topics/answers/2003/ANS01235.html

It refers to the popular **Stamina Rx**", "**Stamina RX for Women**", "Sigra", "Y-Y", "Spontane ES" and "Uroprin". The problem is a prescription-strength drug, which has not been labeled. It can interact with several other drugs, which people with erectile dysfunction often use and the result is a dangerous lowering of the blood pressure, which **can trigger a stroke**! The FDA's Office of Criminal Investigations has already launched an investigation of the case.

This example shows that even if you are well familiar with the ingredients of such supplements, there is a **great risk** to contain **illegal substances.** Just imagine that you take such pills convinced that they will improve your sexual life and instead of this, a <u>stroke puts an end to your life</u> for "only 49.95"! After I learnt about such incidents resulting from **6 different pills,** my confidence in these supplements vanished completely.

One very common herb used in sex and penis enlargement pills is **yohimbe**. FDA warns that it has serious adverse effects especially when taken with <u>cheese, liver and red wine</u>. Overdosing can cause even **death**! For more information visit FDA's "Illnesses and Injuries Associated with Selected Dietary Supplements" at <u>www.cfsan.fda.gov/~dms/ds-ill.html</u>

While yohimbe is dangerous mainly in high doses or due to interactions, there is another potentially deadly substance- "**L-Dopa**". From biochemical point of view, this is amino acid, which is the exact precursor of Dopamine in your body. L-Tyrosine, which you are already familiar with, has to go through 3 stages including L-Dopa before it finally converts into Dopamine. However, the difference in the safety profiles of these two amino acids is **huge**. What do I mean? I know of at least 4 clinical references about <u>potential carcinogenic effect of L-Dopa</u>!

1. McGregor DB, Riach CG, Brown A, *et al Environ Mol. Mutagen* 11(4):523-544, 1988
2. Martinez A, Urious A, Blanco M. ***Mutat Res*** 467(1):41-53, 2000
3. Glatt H ***Mutat Res*** 238(3):235-243, 1990
4. Suter W, Matter-Jaerger I ***Mutat res*** 137(1):17-28, 1984

Every time when a new penis enlargement/sex pill or Human Growth Hormone Secretagogue pops up on the market and I see L-Dopa among the ingredients, I become mad. For me this simply means one more product, which has the clinically proven potential to increase the number of **diagnosed cancer and death**.

Every year when I review the statistics and forecasts about cancer, strokes, AIDS, depression and suicides, I feel very bad because **at least 50%** of the men are in their 20s and 30s.

Yes, it is true that the **safe L-tyrosine** will need some time to convert into Dopamine. But it does not matter if you win some time, if you develop cancer in the end and eventually <u>lose your life</u>. Millions of men do **not** know these facts and many others. However you already have a choice. Make your decisions wisely about **L-Dopa** and all other harmful substances exposed in the book!

Learn from the Mistakes of the Porn Stars

If you have some idea about porn movies have you noticed the condition of the men's penises? Their bodies usually are good looking and athletic. However, if the actors have serious deficiencies of vital substances, it takes them much longer to get an erection. Furthermore, it is less then rock hard and up-right.

Then have you paid attention to the sex positions used in most of the porn movies? They are exactly those, which couples should **avoid.** They provide **minimum** stimulation for her, while giving him **maximum** stimulation to maintain hard erection a longer time. If their bodies and sexual systems are fully loaded with all key substances for ultimate performance and abilities, it should be **exactly the opposite**.

Men should have **very sensitive** penises (local parasympathetic nerves loaded with acetylcholine) and hard, massive and upright erection. Only then will it continuously stimulate the vagina's upper most sensitive line. The only thing, which is still needed, is long-lasting ejaculation control. To achieve this, it is definitely **not** a good idea to use sex positions, which specifically trigger the entire front part of a penis and its upper most sensitive spot.

Men from porn movies have sex for a living. You can have them as an example **what exactly happens** when you leave your body to manage on itself and regularly put on it great sexual or physical pressure.

Have you ever wondered how at least 50% of these men can maintain great intensity of the thrusts without blowing off for some time? The answer is in their (**severe**) **Acetylcholine deficiency**. A penis, which points downwards, shows completely shut down local parasympathetic nervous functions. The first result from this is **sexual insensitivity** and **locked production** of NO and cGMP. This is the reason why their penises are often horizontal or hang downwards even after an intensive oral stimulation and sex.

Deficiency of Acetylcholine automatically means also **sluggish work of the liver.** It has to supply the 5-alpha-reductaze enzyme for the conversion of testosterone into DHT. This is the reason why sometimes their penises are less than rock hard even at the time of ejaculation. Then they often just **ooze out few drops**, which is not impressive at all. It is usually almost clear liquid, which also means very low concentration of sperm. Here are the reasons for all these chronic problems:

- deficiency of water
- deficiency of Acetylcholine
- deficiency of Dopamine
- deficiency of L-Arginine/HGH
- deficiency of Prostaglandin E-1

I find it amusing when I see an ad in a magazine or news-paper for yet another sex pill, which pledge to "double" your ejaculation volume. In order to achieve it you don't have to buy $50-$70 fancy herbal pills.

Normal ejaculation produces about 3 cc (3 ml) of semen. The sperm makes up less than 1% of the volume while the prostate creates about 25% and the seminal vesicles about 70%. The sperm has extremely high concentra-tion of PGE-1, zinc, potassium, fructose and citric acid. There are also many other little known substances in the semen.

Add to all this the observation of the ancient sex mas-ters in China, according to whom the vital energy in your sperm is more than 50% of the available in your body! Because of all these, I strongly recommend that you lick/ drink it after ejaculation. In this way, great amounts of sev-eral important minerals and especially prostaglandin will return to your body. If the ancient Chinese manuscripts are accurate, this will return most of the expended vital energy as well.

In the past I never paid attention to it. The problem after that was fatigue and especially some cold feeling inside my body. The conversion of Serotonin into Melatonin ex-plains the drowsiness. However, according to the ancient masters, your sperm is "yang" or **hot** and once you shoot it out, the dominant energy left in you is the remaining "yin" or **cool** one.

Under appropriate conditions, your sperm can create a new human being. I will take this concept one step further with the fact that if there were enough women for each of the spermatozoids in your semen, you could become the father of 300 million people from just 1 ejaculation! We can only imagine what incredible amount of energy we release/sacrifice from our bodies for a new life.

Then, wouldn't it be better if you do **not** ejaculate without intending to create a child? Unfortunately, men **have to** ejaculate and I have already provided the optimal frequency for each age group. The reason is the negative testosterone feedback in the body. If your testicles are not emptied regularly, they will slow down the production of sperm <u>and testosterone</u>. The more you are sexually passive, the lower will drop your testosterone levels with all the consequences.

Do you want to <u>triple</u> your ejaculation volume? If your answer is positive, just follow the free/cheap and 100% science-based principles for ultimate sexual performance and health presented in the book. Once the few major factors, substances and organs are the way they should be, everything else will **automatically** improve and increase. Particularly important for significant ejaculation volume are:

- water
- Arginine
- Zinc
- Folic acid

If you are in your 30s and ooze out several drops of sperm at 1-2 inches, expect to start shooting at **more than 1**

meter quantities equal to **2-3 table spoons**. This can increase **3-5 times your ejaculation volume**. Expensive pills can hardly beat the significant increase you can get by simply drinking **2-3 liters** of water. If you consider it "too much", the FDA's daily recommended intake of water for men above 19 years is 3.7 liters. Start with 2 liters and you will notice the difference in your ejaculation volume.

If you wonder why water is the most important factor just think for a while. A highly concentrated sperm is quite heavy and drops down immediately. On the contrary, highly diluted sperm, which consists mainly of water, is very light and can easily "fly" at a long distance. To sum up, the more water in your sperm, the greater the total quantity you will ejaculate at a greater distance. However, not all men will like watery ejaculations. If you want greater fertility or density, you can use several **Chinese herbs**. You can find them in the Directory of Vital Substances.

Learn from Impotent Men

Imagine a wild lion, which has…, erectile dysfunction. It sounds funny to me. However, there are more than **30 million** representatives of male Homo Sapiens only in the USA, who are **completely impotent**. A recent survey of Reuters Health conducted in the UK among impotent men shows that

- 50% report low self confidence
- 25% are embarrassed to discuss it even with their wives
- 14% have suicidal thoughts
- 14% report affected family life
- 6% report relationship break-ups
- 44% suffer from depression (The Impotence Association)

- many wait for years before seeking treatment

You already know what the reasons for premature ejaculation and erectile dysfunction (impotence) are. Each one of them can easily vanish if you focus on your body and everything it needs in order to function properly.

For more than 3 million years, our ancestors neither had had access to pharmaceutical products nor had died with millions from cancer, diabetes, obesity, stroke, etc. They had lived close to Mother Nature having to eat only moderate amounts of simple natural food.

The Dark Side of Viagra and Cialis

Viagra and Cialis state in their fine prints that their pills can cause several **serious side effects, including blindness,** investigated by FDA. Furthermore, the fact that they have been on the market for years and the number of impotent men **only increases** with every year shows that they do nothing to permanently solve this problem!

I am also familiar with business operations and I know that big companies simply do **not** have financial interest to offer you a permanent solution because large profits come from continued sales. No wonder that both drug manufacturers state that they do **not** cure erectile dysfunction. This clearly shows that if you want to have an erection, sensitivity, volume, etc. you have to buy some expensive pills **repeatedly**.

That's why if you hear or read for yet another fancy and expensive pill, gadget or exercise just **skip them**. If it is expensive and does not permanently solve your problem, then you do **NOT** need it! Even drugs approved by the FDA can never substitute the role of your genital parasympathetic nerves, 5-alpha-reductaze from your liver, NO/cGMP or some other naturally occurring substances in the male body.

I wonder how millions of men can pay **$49.95** for only **4** Viagra 100 mg pills or **$99 for only 4 Cialis 10mg pills**. It will pay off much better if you invest this money in your sexual and overall health. With $99, you can buy nearly 500 capsules of the very best multi-vitamin/mineral formula in the world or 1250-1625 top quality capsules, containing **all amino acids** derived from natural whey protein.

Talking about famous erectile drugs, I went to the official web site of Cialis and tried to look at it through the eyes of an average man with very limited biochemical knowledge. I read the "How it works" section and this question was the last one they were concerned to answer. I learnt from another site that the drug targets the PDE-5 (Phospho-de-esterase type 5) enzyme. They are yet another multi-million pharmaceutical giant, which does **not** even bother to tell you what the mechanism of action of their drug is.

From their extremely superficial site I got the impression that all they want you to do is pay, put the pill in your mouth and be thankful for having some erection. It is obvious that they do **not** want you to think, know or ask about in-depth information. Also, due to the possible side effects of this "FDA approved" drug, you may end up having serious problems.

The appearance of Cialis made me very concerned because its effect lasts longer than that of Viagra. Men with mild erectile dysfunction can easily get **Priapism** (erection lasting more than 2-3 hours). Even the company has warned that this condition "must be treated as soon as possible or lasting damage can happen to your penis <u>including the inability to have erections</u>." Can you imagine? You pay for several incredibly expensive pills and as a result, you end up **irreversibly impotent!**

The reason is hidden in the mechanism of action of both Cialis and Viagra. They prevent the release of the PDE-5 enzyme, whose role is to destroy cGMP and as a result your erection will disappear. However, if you have non-stop erection for hours then the blood can flow neither in nor out. The death of the penis is a result from the cut-off supply of Oxygen. That's why **NEVER** take Viagra, Cialis or some other drug for erectile dysfunction <u>without really having such problem.</u>

Learn from Uncommunicative Fathers and Impotent Teenagers Who Commit Suicide

I know about many young men who have tried Viagra before having sex for the first time without having erectile problems and the result was **severe Priapism**. After the erection lasted for several hours, their penises were **permanently damaged**. These men become <u>irreversibly impotent</u> right after the start.

This only proves why it is **extremely important** for mature men/fathers to **pass** such knowledge and experience on teenagers and adolescents. Are you a father of a teenager? There is a good possibility that your son is one of those young men who become <u>permanently impotent</u> because of Priapism, pills, illegal drugs, over-masturbation/ejaculation, etc.

I think the greatest tragedy for a father is to watch how his son becomes more and more closed and depressed for no obvious reason and to have no idea what the reasons might be. Imagine how **you** would feel if you became irreversibly impotent after your first intercourse! Being sexually capable is important for mature men. However, after many years of sexual activity and having children, any problems in this direction are not that catastrophic.

That's why only 14% of the men in Reuter's survey have reported suicidal thoughts. However, when it comes to teenagers, the situation is completely different. According to official report presented at the BBC Health News, **"20% of all deaths by young people are by suicide."** By reading numerous statistics about teen suicides and reading posts at forums, I can confidently say that at least 50% of the impotent teenagers have serious intentions about a suicide.

The second problem is that in contrast to mature men, teenagers **do commit suicides**. The alarming message from the statistics is that the number of suicides is on the **increase!** I can hardly think of a better reason for a teen's suicide than painful irreversible impotence right after their first intercourse.

That's why I have declared war to fathers who do nothing and will use statistics and facts to wake them up and convince them to take action today! It is true that my main objective in this book is **your** ultimate sexual performance and health. However, the **ultimate sexual health of your son(s)** is my target as well. If I do my job properly, I will severely disturb the composure of those fathers, who do not want to talk at least once with their son(s) about sexual education. Nowadays, this can easily lead to a **family catastrophe**.

There is a common illusion among fathers that "your boy" is still a boy. I will not be surprised if he starts having sex from the age of 14. Think about the following situation.

You achieve outstanding sexual abilities, performance and health, while your teen son becomes impotent and commit suicide? If you want to use some lame excuse that such events happen with "**other**" fathers and their sons, please **don't**! It is **high time** I hope you realized. These statistics are **not** about some imaginary people but about real people like **you and your son(s).**

That's why as a father you must provide a **solid sexual education** to your son. It has to protect him from temporary or permanent damages and sexually transmitted diseases including **AIDS**. Otherwise, **you will fail as a father.** I prefer to be painfully honest and straightforward. I'd rather you were angry with me and even hated me instead of finding yourself one day at **your son's funeral** and hating yourself for the rest of your life! Once again, **forget about "other" people**. There is only you and your son.

If I have a child, I will definitely **not** wait for them to become 15-20 years old to start their sexual education. It is easier to start slowly from the age of 2.5-3 and gradually build upon this foundation. However, what would I do if I had an already grown up teenager? Well, there is a "hard" and a "smart" way. Regarding the first one, when I start to talk, even if words fail me, I will continue to talk, because the sexual education of my son is my personal responsibility and duty. It is **NOT a job of the porn industry!**

However, I know that even a small talk about sex can lay a huge stress on the average father. I definitely do **not** want you to get a heart attack by doing it. That's why here is a **useful plan** how to become one of **the top 1% awesome fathers.**

After you have read the book, put a piece of paper or some other mark **10 pages** before the end of the book. Then leave it with its **front cover up** at a place where your son can see it and make sure that he has indeed seen it. On the next day leave it at the end of a shelf with other books and forget about it for a few weeks. You can be **100% sure** that the teen's irresistible curiosity about sex will make him read it from cover to cover.

Well, it would be even better if you **give it to him**. A third win-win option is to **leave it under his pillow**. If you want to use some special occasion, the most appropriate day would be his 14th birthday. Regardless of the way you choose, he will receive **A-Z knowledge** on how to achieve and maintain ultimate sexual health, performance and abilities. And he will know that he owes it to **you**- his awesome, caring for his sexuality, long life and well-being father. If you have made it that far, there is one more extremely important thing he has to receive from you. I will share it a little bit later. Then he will reasonably consider you in **top 0.1% of all fathers**.

Little Known Statistics and Stories Every Father and Teenager Should Know

There is a "smart" way to overcome a <u>deadly threat</u> you should know about. Recently I had a chat with a conservative father online. At one time, we hit the red-hot level:

- My father died from stroke when I was 18. He had never told me anything about sexual education and had hugged me less than 5 times. Why the hell should I sweat and get heart palpitations just from the thought of talking about sex with my 16-year-old son?
- Because you have the chance to **prove yourself better than your father**. Do you think that he did not want to talk

with you about sex? Do you think it was easy for him to play the "Tough Man"- cold, serious and distanced? Now you can understand how **he** was feeling. I don't think that you should judge him for **not** being confident enough to talk with you just like 99% of all fathers. However, there is a world of difference between the situation from your teens and the world **now** in which your son grows.

I sent him the following information and a few stories. In 2003, young people (**15-24**) accounted for **50% of all new HIV infections worldwide!**

6,000 children and adolescents become infected with HIV every day!

In 2004, there were **2.2 Million HIV positive people under 15!**

Source: report of **WHO,** December, 2004 (World Health Organization)

Estimated HIV/AIDS diagnoses in the US 2000-2003

15-24 **12%   37,599**
25-34 **27%   311,137**

Estimated AIDS deaths in US 1999-2003

15-24 **9,789**
25-34 **142,761**

Source: US Department of Health and Human Services, Centers for Disease Control and Prevention (CDC)

Here are few extracts of teenagers' touching stories sent to **www.Avert.org**, a leading AIDS charity, which is an incredibly valuable site for young people.

Monica: "I am 15 years old, my best friend who is a male has AIDS, and we were really close. So one night we experimented and **after** the fact that we "did it", he told me that he had AIDS. I was so angry at him and scared. I told my mom and she took me to be tested right away. Unfortunately, I was HIV positive. I went in my room and cried for days…"

Sophie: "I am not very sure how I came to get the virus. When I had my test, one of my **ex-boyfriends** had just died in an accident. So maybe he had the virus and **didn't know it**, I don't know."

Paul: "I found out that I had HIV in 1991. I believe I got the infection from an **ex-girlfriend** who I now know slept around during our relationship. During this time **I was only sixteen**."

Matt: "I knew I'd been unsafe a couple of times but I really thought the **odds were in my favour**. I felt well, happy, and very much alive. On January 18th at 10.00 am, I was diagnosed HIV positive. My stomach and heart plunged… I sat on a bench and wondered **how I would tell my partner**… I cried on and off for most of the following week…"

Clara: "My <u>first boyfriend</u> was a guy called Steve. We started to grow apart when we left school, and I started college. Just before my 20th birthday, my parents were diagnosed with cancer and I heard through my friends that Steve had started getting ill. Steve had barely reached **20** and I found myself <u>at his funeral</u>…
One night at a nightclub, Daniel mentioned that his sister had told him that Steve **had died of AIDS**. I snapped back at him. No one knew Steve like I did and <u>he would have told me</u>… Well, three days after the blood test , **my life ended**….I was threatened and judged like I should

have known Steve had AIDS - **I was** only 17 **then for goodness sake. A child, that's all I was.**"

I think that Clara's story is a **superior example** why and how HIV/AIDS spreads like a wild fire around the world. In most cases, it comes from a very close boy/girlfriend, which looks perfectly healthy. It usually **takes them years** to learn that they have the deadly virus. By that time **all** their intimate partners are already infected! As you can see from these true stories, they were **12-17** years old when they got the fatal disease.

Clara, **doomed to die soon** and one of more than **2.2 million** infected children, tragically concludes: "A child, that's all I was". Those **151,000 teenagers and adolescents** who have **died** of AIDS in the last few years only in the USA could still be alive. I am 100% sure. If their parents had taken action and provided them with a solid sexual education, a great part of those lives could have been spared. But they had thought that such things happen only with **"others"** and have found themselves **at the funeral of their children!**

You can **not** stop your children to have sex. It is only a matter of when and with whom. Steve had known perfectly well about his disease BUT did **not** tell Clara before it was **too late**. Can we judge him, a 17-year-old teenager? I think that it is wiser to learn from these mistakes and make sure it will **NOT** happen with **your children**.

The extremely high levels of testosterone in the men at this age force 98% of them to have sex. At such moments, rational thoughts are left behind. That's why it is a doomed battle for parents who try to stop their children from having sex or rely that they will stop themselves. There are 3 hierarchically produced substances in the brain of a young man. The more he does **not** obey to the inner sexual rush, the higher ranking and therefore stronger substance is released. Their accumulated peak will lead to a kind of **rational blackout and sexual obsession**.

This is the biochemical reason behind the shocking results in a report by the family therapist Dr. Judith Majors Avis. According to it, **25%** of the men studying in a college have made a **forced intercourse** with an unwilling partner! However, the most horrific result she reported was that **20%** of the male college students say that they **would rape a woman** if they have a guarantee that they will not be exposed and punished! Some part of the women has been infected with HIV exactly as a result from a **rape**.

At the age of 18 I personally refused to obey to the nature's rush to have sex. It is very difficult to describe the **incredible struggle and agony** I went through. Very few men will even think to fight especially when they have close female friends like Clara who want to "experiment". This once again puts the emphasis on **promoting safe sex** instead of preaching moral.

I remember clearly a dialog with a Supervisor from my past who told me once: "I never give unwanted advice or suggestions. Instead I build a **strong relationship** with each of my people and make it clear that my door is always open for anything whatsoever." I don't know about the others but personally, I have gone to him **many, many times** asking about anything. He is one of the very few people I have talked with about sex and women. He is a perfect example of a **leader** who <u>leads by example</u> and is really of great help and value for the people around him. I believe that every parent should be like him.

Now let's go back to the reaction of that conservative father online, which surprised me. Here is what he wrote to me. "Especially these children's stories moved me to tears. Shit! I am a stupid, ignorant and blind for the deadly reality man just like my father! I will print out these statistics and stories. Then I will go to buy a box of condoms. After my son come back from school and read these materials, I will put his hand on the big Bible. Then I will ask him to swear that no matter with whom, when or where he has sex, he will always think first for the safety of his partner and himself and use condoms! I prefer to get a stroke while making sure that my son will live long enough, instead of at the moment I learn that he has AIDS." (or commit suicide after he becomes permanently impotent)

The Solution to the Embarrassment when Purchasing Condoms

I know that when it comes to condoms many people feel embarrassed. That's why I made an experiment trying to find out a "smart" solution to this crucial for the prevention of AIDS issue. I bought **50 boxes** of top quality condoms from the biggest mall. When buying such quantities, they think that I have a shop and no one cares at all. I opened **5 boxes** and put **20 condoms** at a few strategic places all over my house. Then I invited all my friends. For the next 7 days 52 people passed through my house. Most of them were friends coming with their friends. I was maintaining every day about **20 available condoms**.

The first thing, which everyone noticed were the condoms. The official version was: "I am fed up with **not** having a condom nearby when I need one. That's why if you don't have, take as much as you want." In such friendly environment and with a very "generous" owner of **abundant quantity** of condoms, people were really taking directly or secretly.

At the end of the week, I made a calculation and was astonished by the result. The number of condoms, which were missing, was equal to **20 boxes**. This showed that each visitor in the age range from 19-32 had taken approximately **4 condoms** in just 1 week. The reason can be a real need, rare opportunities to get condoms or both.

For the following 3 weeks, I kept on maintaining 5 boxes and 20 spread condoms in my house. Without calling anyone anymore, I noticed a **300% increase** in the frequency of friends' visits. The number of disappearing condoms remained relatively the same. After the end of that month, I stopped the experiment and waited to see what will happen. Those already 92 people were obviously not pleased with the change. I started probing: "After all, we can buy condoms from so many places. What is the problem to buy few at a time?" The reaction was: "Well, you know that the **feeling** is not that comfortable."

If buying a condom is **not** something adults can deal with easily, then imagine **how teenagers feel**. At the end they have almost no other choice but to believe, just like Matt, that the "odds were in my favour". That's why I think that such indirect approach as my experiment can be **especially helpful** for young teenagers and adults in a family. All that parents have to do is **keep about 10 condoms** at several places in your bedroom.

In this way whenever your son/daughter needs a condom, it will be easy to take one of the available. If you use condoms to avoid pregnancy, instead of secretly throwing them, put them in the trash bin. After all, you have to give your children an **example** that condoms are **not for decoration** but you really **use them**.

The last thing they should know is to avoid oral sex. This is the other major way you can get the HIV virus in addition to vaginal sex without a condom. Of course, using a used hypodermic needle for injecting (illegal) drugs is the third way to catch HIV.

I included this "common" topic because I work with exact facts and figures. This means that you/your son should know from **A-Z** how to avoid AIDS. If you know only **one thing**, such as using a condom, **but** make unsafe oral sex with an infected woman, the result will be the same- **infection and death**.

The Ultimate "Smart" Plan for Teen's Sex Education, Penis Enlargement and the Father's Role in it

During the night, your body produces **maximum levels** of Human Growth hormone and testosterone. That's why the best time for penis enlargement and sex is when you wake up in the morning. Whether you have a partner or not is not that important. However, I want to underline that masturbation and sex exert **different levels of influence** on your body.

Masturbation (manual stimulation of your penis) is appropriate to boost your testosterone levels or release the produced sperm in your testicles. I want to stress on how **crucial** is to follow strictly the healthy ejaculation frequency. For teenagers 13-19 it is up to 3 times per week and there must be an interval of at least 1 day between them!

On the other side, **sex** has a **profound impact** on your body and stimulates practically **all your glands**. Having sex for at least 10 minutes every single morning plus some sexual activity throughout the day is the **real "fountain of youth"** In addition, it is one of the major factors for optimum health and weight.

The most important thing about your daily sexual activity and penis enlargement is to **avoid ejaculation in the morning**. As you already know, penis enlargement needs high levels of DHT in your penile tissues and the building up of **new** DHT receptors. At the time when you are about to ejaculate, your penis is **fully loaded** with blood rich in DHT, amino acids and all other important substances.

After you ejaculate, you lose erection within minutes and the blood withdraws almost completely from your penis. This immediately **puts an end** to any constructive (penis enlargement) process. That's why if you want to encourage it, take advantage of the morning hours and ejaculate at a different time like afternoon or evening.

For teenagers, stimulating their penis in the morning is almost unavoidable, because of the great sexual excitement generated from the high levels HGH and testosterone. That's why it is a responsibility of every father to know this and use it for the benefit of his son.

Avoiding the morning ejaculations will guarantee him massive penis about **5.5-7 inches in length.** Thus your son will never worry about the size of his penis. Furthermore, the initial enlargement of a man's penis occurs exactly during the early teen years. That's why you have to encourage it **exactly at this period** because after that it is more difficult.

I do believe that it is **high time** fathers and sons **broke the ice** regarding sex and share their experience and knowledge. This will dramatically reduce the mistakes, which lead to temporary or permanent damages of the penis with all the horrible consequences. We live in a world where AIDS and sexually transmitted diseases **reign** and the age to start having sex drops with every year. That's why this situation requires from every single father to <u>take action today</u>! Tomorrow can be too late.

Learn From My Meeting with Death

We all have had those moments when we simply feel down and nothing is able to lift us up. The problem is when you keep on getting closer to the bottom day after day. If I consider myself now a "high-testosterone" man, this is mainly because I came from the extreme of the other side. Till my dying day, a **scar across the veins** will remind me of a more special meeting in my life- the one with **Death**.

During my entire childhood, I was closed and shy with quite anti-social behaviour. Being a brilliant student was **never enough**. I had to be much more. The constant huge demand of parents, teachers and professors was slowly but steadily pushing me downwards. During my late teens, the levels of testosterone normally reached the peak in my life. However, I did **not know how to react** to my everyday erections. No one talked with me about this. The majority of information in Internet was written by deeply religious men who considered it a **"mortal sin"**, which has to be eradicated.

Now I know that due to **over ejaculations,** I had developed a severe deficiency of Dopamine as a result from Serotonin depletion. At the same time huge doses of

Adrenalin were pushing me towards **extreme** "fight or flight" behaviour. Now I am sure that due to its influence combined with the threats in Internet for "going to hell for eternity for my masturbations", my personal classification of self-stimulation gradually became **negative ("sinful").**

Thus my life turned into a **24 hours' hell**. The more I tried to restrict myself, the more I needed to do it. Gradually I **almost stopped eating** just to break the resistance of my body. When even this had no success, I started beating myself because I preferred it to going "to hell for eternity". I reached the point when I was out of my mind with **often blackouts** because of the starvation. At the same time, my mind was locked by anti-natural and fundamentally wrong idea. I will skip the scene when the cold kitchen knife cut my veins. Instead, I want to say what helped me to come back from the point few people have returned from.

I didn't have **even one reason to continue living** in this "sinful, out of control body". However, in my mind there was the radiant smile of my spiritual mother, Dr. Shri Mataji. During my 6 hell-like teen years her amazing love, personal example, "sahaja yoga meditation" and encouragement through lectures gave me optimism and inner strength to continue forward despite everyone and everything. That's why I had **no** right to break her heart by leaving this world. Then I decided that I will stay and **dedicate my life for the people's welfare,** just like her.

Looking back, I can see how right she is that every single person has **tremendous potential inside**, which has to be **awaken** and **developed** for the betterment of yourself and the world as a whole. She has numerous international awards, including a Nobel Prize Nomination for Peace in 1996. In addition to them, I can only offer her my humble and deepest gratitude for being such an **enormous source** of motivation and inspiration for millions of people all over the world. With this book and the next ones, I want to prove to myself that I have learnt something from her. Furthermore, I want to become a similar **solid and resourceful foundation** for many people.

Staying alive required from me to find a mental escape. I had **no idea** how I will find a solution to this crisis, but I decided to start eating again and try not to think a lot about the masturbations.

The time was passing and the "Big Four" in a man- **Testosterone, Serotonin, Growth Hormone and Dopamine** increased and normalized my thinking and behaviour. Then some shocking things started to dawn on me. The first one was how **deformed** my image of God was. Instead of an ocean of love, compassion and forgiveness, to me he was just like some merciless, ferocious, fire-breathing demon, which can't wait to see me make even the slightest mistake to give the worst punishment. This **calmed me down.**

Later I was even more shocked to realize, that to please God (stop the "sinful" masturbations) I almost killed myself! **This** was already an <u>unacceptable (sinful) action</u>. He has given me this body and life and it is my responsibility to take **utmost care for them**. This discovery was the light in the tunnel that the whole development and concept for the sinful masturbations was **fundamentally wrong.**

I started going to kinder gartens, watching how parents interact and behave with their children. The only thing I was seeing over and over again, was **enormous love, care and understanding**. If God is my Creator, he should be **no different**. This whole story formed in a unique way my relationship with God. I made a promise to never again let some human ideas stand between us and interfere with the **natural processes and outcomes** in my body and life. I also realized that I knew **little** about the way the human, and especially male body, functions. The result from this was **almost fatal** for me.

This sparked my insatiable pursuit of A-Z knowledge in this area. What I gradually learnt was 100% back up of my conclusions. The testicles produce **sperm 24 hours a day**, which on a regular basis **must** be released through ejaculations. If it is not done consciously, <u>the body will do it</u> during a man's sleep. The strong connection between the level of sexual activity and production of testosterone is also of **great importance**. If I see an obese man, I'd bet that his overall sexual activity is **low.** That's why daily sexual activity is **one of the key points** for achieving and maintaining <u>optimum weight and health</u> in "Your Scientific Diet for Men".

I gradually **freed myself from any guilt or illusions** regarding masturbations. When I need to do it (to boost my testosterone levels) I am calm that God, like a **loving and understanding father** knows and is happy that I do something <u>good for my body</u> which also makes me feel great and uplifted. Every man knows that it is quite tough to find a girlfriend and especially to get married. That's why for many years we have to manage somehow. I am 100% sure that God prefers us to masturbate, instead of to fuck bitches.

I have experienced first hand what is to have **extremely low** testosterone, dopamine, serotonin and growth hormone levels. At the same time, being under the absolute dominance of **Adrenalin** and **Cortisol** nearly killed me! In my case, it became <u>self-destructive</u>. For other people this can lead to (shocking) crimes. I hope that you now understand why I will <u>never again allow </u>a serious drop in the "Big Four" in my body.

Looking towards the future, I can predict that more stress and pressure will be laid on men all over the world. This makes it even more important to **support and encourage one another** to keep our heads above the water. I know that it is not easy and that it requires a lot of efforts and even struggle. It is very easy to get depressed, pessimistic and **automatically slash your "Big Four".** Yes, but is this "life"? Are you of benefit to yourself and the world around you? Here is a great quote from a legendary manager:

"Motivation is everything. You can do the work of two people, but you **can't** be two people. Instead, you have to **inspire the next guy down the line and get him to inspire his people.**" by Lee Iacocca.

During my life and practice of "sahaja yoga meditation", I have realized that there are **no "bad"** people. There are only people with certain problems who badly need loving, understanding and empathizing attitude. It is **never easy** to be bad and to hurt the others.

If we distance ourselves from <u>superficial things</u> such as colour, nationality, race, etc. we **all** have sensitive hearts and souls. We **all** need love, attention and appreciation from the others. Once I realized it and generously started giving them to the people around me, I witnessed a **tremendous increase** of love, attention and recognition towards me!

You, as a man, always make the first step. **You** demonstrate high "emotional intelligence" by being generous in compliments, recognition, listening, assisting and staying tuned to the needs of all those around you. The rest (towards you) simply follow. Dr. Shri Mataji has said it very well: "Open the door of receiving. Then open the door of giving and enjoy the circulation between them."

We live in a world, which is almost suffocated by **stress and fear.** That's why **we, men,** have more opportunities to do unlimited number of activities than ever before. They can easily boost our testosterone levels as well as contribute to the betterment of the world. I am deeply thankful for this **golden opportunity** and use it every single day.

"Look at a day when you are supremely satisfied at the end. It's not a day when you lounge around doing nothing; it's when you had everything to do, and you have done it." by Margaret Thatcher

I have always wondered what I can do to change this world. Few years ago, a friend of mine wrote to me a thank-you card, which to my great surprise gave me the answer. "**By changing yourself you have already changed the world.**" It is so true. You are an important part and particle of this world. That's why you hold a piece of its opportunity to change for better. I do hope that you will use it and will contribute to a **happier, safer and better world.** And I know one thing, which will skyrocket your sexual pleasure and life. This is the knowledge for **The VIP Muscle®.**

The VIP Muscle- Men's Multi-Orgasms Generator

Read this chapter <u>only after</u> you have read and applied the information presented so far. Without loading your body at least with lecithin/choline, your VIP Muscle will **not work properly!** That's why the first step you have to take is to prepare your body.

The best time for dealing with this little known muscle is after you wake up in the morning. First, go to the bathroom because <u>your bladder must be empty!</u> The reason is that you use the so called PC (Dr. Kegel's tailbone or pubococcygeus) muscle to stop/hold your urine. The VIP Muscle is near to the PC muscle. The most important thing about these two muscles is that they function **opposite to each other**. The **PC** is directly connected with your **Sympathetic nervous system**. In addition, it is directly responsible for the <u>ejaculation instinct and process</u>.

On the contrary, the **VIP Muscle** is connected with your **Parasympathetic nervous system**, which is responsible at a sexual level for the powering and long sustaining of your erection. That's why if you contract even few times your PC muscle during masturbation or sex this will <u>immediately activate</u> your local sympathetic nerves.

The result is usually **premature ejaculation!** That's why from now on contract it **only** to stop peeing or to push the last few drops of urine and for nothing else! This is the first and most important step towards **outstanding sexual endurance!** It is a <u>fundamentally wrong</u> myth that by contracting the PC muscle you can delay or hold the instinctive process of ejaculation. It may work for few seconds or minutes before you finish.

Step-By-Step How to find out the VIP Muscle

The PC and the VIP Muscle are situated at the two sides of your anus. The **PC is right below your testicles.** It is bigger in size and is easily noticeable on touch. The VIP Muscle is **exactly below your tail bone** at the base of your spinal cord. To make it easier for you, follow the following steps to find it out.

1. After you wake up, go to the bathroom and then go back to your bed. Stand on your knees and spread them a little bit.
2. Let your butt touch your heels. Use them to open gently its two halves around 1" (2.5 cm) aside. This will stretch a little bit the PC and VIP muscles and make them more accessible and distinguishable.
3. With your preferred hand for masturbation, hold tightly your penis. Start slowly moving the index finger of your other hand from the hard on touch tail bone down towards your anus. The VIP Muscle is situated exactly at these <u>2 inches</u>. Put the tips of your fingers on it and start contracting this area until you feel the pulsating muscle.
4. With the fingers of your other hand stroke up and down your penis. Pay special attention to stimulate its "hot spot" which is at the front side exactly below the

head. Usually the middle part of your index finger is on it during masturbation.

5. **Synchronize the strokes with the contractions of the VIP Muscle and flatten your abdominals!** These are the 2 **crucial** requirements to start highly pleasurable contractions. Once again, there should be **no deficiencies** of vital substances in your body.

The Role of the VIP Muscle

Every time you contract the VIP Muscle, you activate the parasympathetic nerves in your genital area. This counteracts with the increasing activation from sexual stimulation of the **sympathetic nerves towards ejaculation**. In addition, this ensures **continuous production of NO/ cGMP**, which powers up and sustains your erection. Of course, you should have prepared your body by loading it with sufficient quantities of

- Choline/Lecithin
- Vitamins
- Minerals
- L-Arginine and L-Tyrosine if necessary

It is true that the VIP Muscle is quite far from your penis. However, even several contractions will quickly generate a **hard and long-lasting erection**. The reason is exactly the strong stimulation of the **local parasympathetic nerves** and the dependent on them production of NO/cGMP.

The VIP Muscle is also the place where the parasympathetic nerves from the front and backside of your genital area connects with the spinal cord and through it with the brain. By stroking your penis or having sex, your body generates pleasure (nerve) signals, which have to go up to the Centre of Pleasure in your brain. Since your genital area is fully loaded with Acetylcholine, millions of powerful and clear signals pass every second through the VIP Muscle. Each contraction serves as a **magnifying glass** and the result is a highly focused feeling of great pleasure. When the contractions become powerful and numerous, they turn into **orgasms.** Then you can easily enjoy 15 per minute.

However, they are concentrated in your tailbone. That's why standing on your knees is good mainly for initial practice until you find and establish a mental connection with this small area.

2 Ways to Intensify the Orgasms

There are several things, which affect **substantially** the intensity and pleasure from the orgasmic contractions. The first thing is **which specific part** of the VIP Muscle is actually contracting. Since this is a large muscle, I recognize **three parts** of it.

1. Lower part- located **next to your anus**. At the beginning, there is a risk to contract the PC muscle instead of the VIP Muscle. The easiest way to make sure that you deal with the right muscle is to **make the following small test**. Contract each of them while you urinate. If you stop or the flow is seriously affected then you have contracted the **PC muscle.** If the contractions do **not** have any serious influence on the current then you have contracted the VIP Muscle.

Note that both muscles are **interconnected**. It is **not** possible to separate them completely. When you stand on your feet it is of great importance towards which of them you will direct your attention. This will mainly determine where the contractions will occur. The lower part is closest to the PC muscle. That's why I do **not recommend** that you attempt to contract it.

2. <u>Middle part</u>- located at the lower angle of the triangular tailbone. Usually this is where I aim to generate contractions because the sensations are incredibly powerful. In addition, it is easy to achieve stronger contractions in this part.

3. <u>Upper part</u>- located right below the spinal cord. The contractions are very small and subtle. However, the pleasurable signals go directly to the brain. Sometimes even the thought about the orgasms from this part make me shiver for a second. They are **extremely powerful** and sometimes **overwhelming!** That's why it is a good idea to be careful with them.

The great pleasurable feelings from contractions in the **middle part** result in **local orgasms**. However, you will notice that the contractions at the **upper part** are quite different. For example, their number can go up to <u>50 per minute</u>. Second, this part of the VIP Muscle is **richest in nerves**. Third, it is the smallest and that's why usually I can feel how **all** generated pleasurable signals "pass" through it towards the brain. The result from all this is a euphoric feeling and I often loose control for a while. However, to achieve significant number of powerful contractions, it is very important the **position of your body.**

3 Positions for the Ultimate VIP Experience

Here are 3 specific positions you can use lying on your bed.

The Mountain Peaks Position

This is **absolutely the best position** for enjoying an out-of-this-world multi-orgasmic experience using the VIP Muscle. Lie on your back and raise your knees up while your feet remain on the bed. Position your legs a little bit wider than your shoulders just **like the letter V**. Make sure that your corps and thighs form a <u>straight angle</u> like the **letter L**.

I have found out that an <u>essential requirement</u> for turning the contractions of the VIP Muscle from pleasurable into orgasmic is to **flatten your lower abdominal muscles and keep them like that!** To get the ultimate from this position, it is also crucial to <u>maintain the straight angle</u> between your thighs and body. You may put a **small pillow** or something else below your feet. Otherwise, if you strain the upper part of your thighs you will get a painful muscle fever later on.

Once you are set, simply stimulate **rhythmically** your penis and **synchronize with it** the contractions of the middle or upper part of the VIP Muscle. Experiment first with one of them and then with the other. There is a great difference in the feeling and that's why I change them regularly during a session.

Caution! You will get a **muscle fever** if you contract the VIP Muscle too many times. That's why begin with a **small number of contractions** and increase them gradually. Allow this small muscle at least 1 week to strengthen and improve its stamina with each "**sexual workout**". Within

2-3 weeks, it will become strong enough and you will be able to generate **powerful and numerous** contractions/ orgasms.

Furthermore, you have to <u>plan your choline/lecithin intake</u> in accordance with the number of times you use the VIP Muscle, because it uses a **significant amount** of Acetylcholine. I contract it many times especially in the morning. That's why instead of 550 mg, I take **1-1.2 g of choline/day** from a supplement. In this way, both my multi-orgasmic activity and Parasympathetic nervous system run perfectly.

The Butterfly Position

This position is a little bit controversial, because it more easily generates contractions of the **PC muscle** instead of the VIP Muscle. However, in the long-term it is very important to **feel precisely** when you activate the PC muscle and your sympathetic/ejaculation mechanism and when your parasympathetic/VIP Muscle.

Again lie on your back and let your feet touch each other. Pull them towards your body and let your knees point left and right. Your legs should be in the following position- <> just like the wings of a butterfly. **Flatten your abdominals**, try to contract your VIP Muscle and notice that it is **not** easy at all. Instead, you have probably contracted your PC muscle, which is right below your testicles. This position is an excellent way to experiment and develop your sense whether you contract the PC or the VIP Muscle. Without this **perfect distinguishing** using the wrong muscle especially during sex will result in **premature ejaculation**.

The Straight Angle Position

This is half "mountain peaks" and half "butterfly" position. Lie on your back and rise up your right knee while your left one is on the bed and points to the left. Your knees should form a straight angle. I like very much this position because you can **achieve both orgasmic contractions** in the middle and upper part of the VIP Muscle.

A Crucial Discovery I Found during a Vacation in Greece

7.16 am- Oh, no! I jumped immediately from my bed, rushed in the bathroom and in just 5 minutes I was driving like crazy to the airport. If I missed the airplane, my vacation would be spoiled. I was lucky enough not to make 2 accidents although I almost crashed in one car just in front of the airport. Thanks God, in the last minute I managed to catch the airplane. Then I had the feeling that something was wrong. **Something important was missing**!

After thinking for a while, I realized that I had **not** taken my multi-vitamin/mineral formula and amino acids. I immediately opened my suitcase and the 2 bottles were indeed missing! Oh, no! What was I going to do? I was upset but then I thought. OK, most of the readers of the book will **not start** with a body fully loaded with the major important substances. This was an excellent opportunity to see what will be the effect on the multiple orgasms, sexual pleasure and my overall condition. For the next 3 days, I did not take any multi formulas and amino acids derived from whey protein.

Already at Greece, I finished with the check in and went for a massage. Then back in the suit, it was time for the experiment. I started with The Mountain Peaks position and in **5 seconds,** I was already enjoying numerous powerful orgasms. I continued for around 5 minutes and stopped because everything was as usual.

On the next day, I also went for a massage and then continued with the VIP Muscle. There was a **difference**! It was **not** as easy to generate many orgasms as the previous day and the level of pleasure was **lower**. Then I was almost sure that taking at least a complete multi formula is simply **critical** for the success of this practice.

On the third day, although I did the same things, the level of the pleasure of the generated contractions was the same as that of the **massage** before that. In fact, I could **not** say that they were "orgasms"! This 3-day experiment proved to me that an advanced multi-vitamin/mineral formula is necessary to enjoy **ultimate** sexual health, abilities and performance.

All vitamins, minerals, amino acids and **choline** are extremely important for the proper functioning of all organs, systems and biochemical reactions in your body. That's why I went in details about the male sexual system and the critical biosubstances, which power and maintain it in top condition. Some of them are so important that I have provided additional in-depth information in the Directory of Vital Substances. Use the information in the book to **identify and eliminate their deficiencies** in your body.

How I aggravated the Crisis after Greece

Once I came back home, I thought that multi formulas and amino acids would be just 2 of **several factors** most of my readers won't have in the beginning. That's why

I decided to **switch to the average lifestyle** and see what will be the result. Therefore, I completely stopped:

- taking Advanced Multi formula
- all Amino acids from whey protein
- GABA before bedtime
- drinking 2.3 liters of water
- avoiding meals after 15.00 o'clock
- walking at least 60 minutes a day

To make the story shorter, here is my condition when I woke up after 4 days. First, I could **not** stop thinking all night. I was semi-conscious although there was nothing to worry about or deserved so much thinking. My **mood was down** and I was worried when I did **not** feel the usual morning erection. This automatically meant that my overall condition was nearing a **depression point**!

The **fastest way** to check my condition was to examine my reactions to sexual arousal. I stimulated my nipples and for my amazement, they were as sensitive as my skin! This automatically meant that my Acetylcholine levels were very low. The penile stimulation for 5 minutes resulted in a **semi-erection!** It was quite soft and the pleasurable sensation was small. Actually, I had **erectile dysfunction and moderate insensitivity**. I tried to generate orgasms through the VIP Muscle but I could **not** even contract it! I was getting more and more anxious and upset.

Then I got up from the bed and for the first time in more than 7 years, I got a **strong pulsating headache** at the back of my head. I thought that probably I have high blood pressure. That's why I measured it for the first time in 3 years. For my astonishment, it was **dangerously low 104/59** as the normal is **120/80**. Furthermore, my blissful radiant and non-stop sense of well-being was **gone**. The problem was that I was already in a **moderate depression**!

While I was passing by a big mirror, I noticed that my waist line is bigger than my hip! I ribbed my eyes because this has **never** happened in my entire life! Once in the bathroom, I looked at the mirror and was shocked. I saw a man with pale dry skin, dark circles below his eyes and looking a few years **older** than what I was used to seeing. I took out a scale from the wardrobe for the first time in 6 years. I had **4.80 pounds** (2.2 kg) above my usual/optimal weight.

I went back to my room feeling very tired and depressed. I could **not** even control my emotions. I dropped down on my knees and almost started crying like a small boy. I thanked God for knowing how exactly to get out of this horrible situation. It was time to **take action** and here is step-by-step **exactly** what I did.

Step-by-Step How I Overcame My Crisis

The first and foremost thing was to drink **17 fl. oz. or 0.5 liter of mineral water.** All those days regarding water I was just like a drug addict dreaming for one more shot. As a result from not more than 3 glasses per day, my throat was all the time as dry as Sahara desert at noon. In **just 15 minutes** when 60% from it was already absorbed **I felt better**.

Then I took **1g of pure choline supplement**, which also contained the necessary amount of Pantothenic Acid for fastest production of Acetylcholine. Due to a severe deficiency of this major neurotransmitter, my erection was gone and my liver could **not** work properly allowing 4.8 extra pounds to stick to my waist line. At 16.00 pm the same day, I took another 1 g of this supplement and by the end of the day, my sensitivity and hard upright erection **were back!**

It was horrible to be in a bad mood and depression. The situation required to use a capsule of **5-HTP**, which is prohibited for prolonged use. Of course, it was pharmaceutical grade! This step was necessary to increase quickly the levels of **Serotonin**. However, I was aware that this definitely would **not** be enough.

When I lifted my hands at the level of the chest, they were **shaking**. This in combination with **obtrusive anxiety** and irrational feeling that something bad will happen, were classical symptoms of **too much Adrenalin**. It had pushed my mind and body in a "Flight or Flight" state. The produced Serotonin from the 5-HTP capsule was going to inhibit the significant conversion of Dopamine into Adrenalin. However, I needed **a lot of Dopamine** to counteract the great quantity of Adrenalin. This was easily achieved by a generous dose of **L-Tyrosine**.

All these major substances require certain vitamins or minerals for optimal and fastest absorption and conversion into other substances. That's why it was high time I took tablets from the very best multi-vitamin/mineral formula. Furthermore, I always take 1-3 tablets with **all 20 amino acids** derived from whey protein soon after the multi formula. They are the **other crucial factor** for the optimal functioning of the human body.

Thus all necessary biosubstances were already inside my body, but still I had another very important thing to do. I had to boost my **testosterone levels**. Since my return from Greece, I almost completely lost any interest towards sexual activity. Thanks God at that time I did **not** have a girlfriend. It was very important to go back to the normal level quickly. It was time to use the almost forbidden combination:

- Bulgarian tribulus terrestris
- Hydroxyandrost-4-ene-6,17-dioxo-3-THP ether (3-OHAT)
- 3,17-diketo-androst-1,4,6-triene (ATD)

Until they affected the testosterone production and levels, I rushed to take 3 of the premium Chinese herbs:

- Schizandra and Lycium Drops
- Siberian Ginseng Drops

I use only 3-5 drops from each one of them on a daily basis, because this is more than enough. However, the crisis justified it to use 20 drops from each. First, I took the Siberian Ginseng. I mixed the drops with a small amount of water and kept it in my mouth for <u>immediate absorption</u> through the tissue below the tongue. Within 2-3 seconds my mind was **cleared** and I felt the typical for it **uplifting** and **overall profound energizing.**

It was turn to the main all-purpose Chinese herb-**Schizandra** combined with **Lycium**. Again within 2-3 seconds while keeping the mixture in my mouth they **completely** pacified, nourished and further energized my whole body, mind and soul. My sense of **blissful and total well-being was back!**

After 30 minutes, I sensed a significant release of **Luteinizing hormone** (LH) from the powerful horny feeling, which filled me up. Very soon after that, my testicles had to produce equally big portions of testosterone. After another 25 minutes, I was absolutely nuts about sex! My testosterone was back to normal and everything was **simply fantastic**. This was a great relieve.

Testosterone itself is a **HUGE** topic and at the same time, a <u>top ranking substance</u>. It is especially important throughout the entire life of a man! The tendency its production to decline with the years is well-known. Moreover, it is a crucial part of the real "**fountain of youth**". That's why I will dedicate a whole chapter to everything related to it in "Your Scientific Diet for Men".

It will include only proven substances, which **naturally boost** directly or indirectly the testosterone production. After that I include reliable ways to minimize its conversion into the female hormone **estrogen**. Constant high levels of testosterone are essential for rock hard erections, optimum weight, lean body and anti-aging.

The market offers hundreds of products and as usually most of them are **little or not effective**. Besides, some of them, especially steroids and pro-hormones, <u>damage severely</u> your testicles, glands and liver and cause significant hair loss. That's why I will cover in full details what works with specific references and what is just fraudulent or harmful for your body.

You already know how to manage with the most common male health problems. However, the biosubstances I have discussed so far have additional, little known benefits. Let's explore them.

Directory of Vital Substances for Ultimate Sexual and Overall Health

In this chapter, I present in full details the information about the majority of those little known and vital biosubstances in your body. As you will see, some of them are quite contradictive. That's why one of my goals is to show you that even looking at multi-vitamin/mineral tablets you can see "vital" substances for your body or very diluted poisons. It is all about the **point of view and knowledge**.

I have included the question: "Are there any side effects?" for each of the discussed substances and the default answer is positive. Take for example Oxygen. It is essential for us. However, in the form of free radicals it is the main reason for our aging and ultimately death.

Actually, there is **not** a substance, which is 100% safe especially at quantities **50-100 times** above the normal intake. That's why it is very important to know the so called "**Toxicity Threshold**" of all substances, vital or not, which you take. By default, my figures are based on the FDA's reports and public warnings. It seems that the

Canadian and EU's equivalent agencies are not interested to invest money simply to rediscover these figures.

Here is a small part of my private **Reference Table of Important Substances**, which has already been discussed in the book. I will present it in its complete form in my next book "Your Scientific Diet for Men".

I personally want "optimal" **and safe** amounts of vitamins, minerals, amino acids, herbs, etc. A quick glance at the Table shows the US RDA (Recommended Daily Allowance) and the Toxicity Threshold of each substance. The "optimal" intake is somewhere in between.

Furthermore, I was shocked when I found two recent research studies, which show that "The Toxicity Threshold" for 2 vital substances is **lower than FDA's figures!** This can be expected as it takes time for FDA's small personnel (10,000) to manage with the huge amount of drugs, foods and supplements and keep themselves updated on the ocean of studies and researches. The problem is that companies rely on their figures and prepare supplements accordingly aiming at "optimal", "ultimate" quantities.

Reference Table of Important Substances

Substances	US RDA	EU RDA
Vitamin B1 (thiamine)	1.1 mg ♀ 1.5 mg ♂	1.4 mg
Niacin (Vitamin B3)	15 mg ♀ 19 mg ♂	18 mg
Pantothenic Acid (Vit.B5)	10 mg	6 mg
Vitamin B6 (pyridoxine)	1.6 mg ♀ 2.0 mg ♂	2 mg
Iron	18 mg ♀ 8 mg ♂	-
Phosphorus	800 mg	800 mg
Zinc	8 mg ♀ 15 mg ♂	15 mg

Substance	Optimal, Safest Dose	FDA's Tolerable Upper Intake	Toxicity Threshold
Vitamin B1 (thiamine)	100 mg	none	150 mg
Niacin (Vit.B3)	150 mg daily total	35 mg (per one intake)	2000 mg
Pantothenic Acid(Vit.B5)	1000 mg	none	none
Vitamin B6	100 mg	100 mg	500 mg
Iron	45 mg	45 mg	not established
Phosphorus	1500 mg	4000 mg	not established
Zinc	15 mg	40 mg	45 mg

Regarding supplements, it is very important to warn you about a little known fact- **toxic impurities**. Nowadays, it is more and more important for companies to keep on reducing the costs in order to stay competitive. However, this means that <u>essential and expensive</u> purifying processes are **not** done. During the production of common supplements such as Vitamin C, **up to 18** purifications must be done. This is necessary because of traditionally used **toxic catalysts** such as arsenic, acetone, lead, hexane, etc. That's why I <u>never buy</u> any supplements which are not clearly labeled "**Pharmaceutical Grade**".

The Federal Pure Food and Drug Act of 1906 is the first to recognize the USP (United States Pharmacopia) as the "official compendia". It gives official status to drugs and other substances set forth in that book. Since that time, the USP has evolved as the official reference book, which sets the standards for the quality and purity of therapeutic agents used in medical practice. Consequently, the USP is utilized by the pharmaceutical industry and the FDA (Food and Drug Administration).

The USP provides assurance to the consumer, as well as those involved in manufacturing and processing, that the quality and purity of the raw materials utilized are of pharmaceutical grade. It is **minimum 98.6% purity** and for certain substances goes to 99.99%.

In this Directory I have provided the standard scientific information with references to journals, researches, books and universities. In all of the studies **only pharmaceutical grade materials** are used. That's why if you want to obtain the same health benefits, you have to take the same pharmaceutical grade nutrients used in them.

Talking about supplements, do you have any idea about the size of this market? In the late 1999, the health-conscious Americans had spent **$15.7 billion** on vitamin, mineral and other supplements! In 2000 the sales were already **$17 billion** and have been on the increase ever since! For comparison, the annual sales of vitamin and nutritional supplements in the UK are around **£400 million** ($763 million).

This ever growing, multi-billion dollar market of supplements is **not** regulated (by FDA). That's why the choice is yours and I would add that the potential problems are also yours. It does **not** make sense to end up with "severe damages up to death" (FDA) from expensive supplement(s) in a pursuit of optimal health, potency and/ or performance.

Take for example the brief overview of all penis enlargement methods. They are simply competing, which will cause you severe and longer-lasting damages. At the same time, they are expensive- $50-$700! That's why let's hunt down for additional harmful or potentially dangerous substances for your health.

The Sweet Aspartame – Deadly Poison or Not

This is the first substance I want to pay very special attention to. Here is a small historical background. For 16 years, FDA has **not** approved of aspartame (50% L-phenylalanine) as a safe substance. What is more, in 1996 it listed **92 symptoms**, from seizures to death, reported in 10,000 consumer complaints. This holds the record for a food additive. Furthermore, the following is an excerpt from Dr. Louis Elsas' testimony recorded in the 8/1/85 Congressional record page S10842:

"**High blood concentrations of L-phenylalanine** are harmful to human brains in at least three situations:

(a) In older than 6 months old children and adults with mature brains high blood concentrations will prolong performance time, slow brain wave cycles (EEG) and reduce neurotransmitter production in a reversible manner.

(b) In newborns to 6 months old with rapidly growing brains elevated blood phenylalanine produces **irreversible brain damage** by slowing migration of oligodendroglia (brain cells) and altering myelin (nerve insulation) formation.

(c) In pregnancy, if the mother's blood phenylalanine is raised in high concentrations, her child's brain development can be **irreversibly damaged**."

That's why if you take any sweeteners such as NutraSweet, have in mind that they contain Aspartame. It comprises of 50% of the amino acid L-phenylalanine. I also want to quote the latest book "Aspartame disease was declared a global epidemic" by Dr. H. J. Roberts. "The Aspartame disease has triggered an avalanche of birth defects and retardation. It releases the tumor agent DKP (diketopiperazine) so **babies** are born with brain tumors. It interferes with their cardiac conduction system causing sudden death".

I found out an interesting study from Sweden regarding methanol, which is a by-product of Aspartame's metabolism. It converts into formaldehyde and formic acid in the body. This is well-known and confirmed by the USA and Canadian Administrations. However, the study has found out that formaldehyde can accumulate in the cells, especially in people with slow metabolism, and cause problems.

However, what FDA and the Movement for Banning of Aspartame agree, is that "High levels of this amino acid in body fluids can cause brain damage."- for reference check (http://www.cfsan.fda.gov/~dms/qa-adf9.html)

That's why FDA has ruled that all products containing aspartame (50% phenylalanine) must specify it on their label. This warning is especially important for **phenylke-tonurics** which genetically lack an enzyme, necessary for the conversion of phenylalanine into a form the body can use.

Despite all these alarming facts, thousands of cases and the latest results from few international researches, the FDA still supports its decision from 1981 that aspartame is **safe**.

Regarding **healthy, non-obese people**, I completely support FDA's position. Some people think that the US FDA is "hiding the truth about this poison" That's why I want to state the position of its <u>Canadian equivalent</u>. Have in mind that it has also approved of aspartame as **safe.** Here is what they have officially written.

"**Allegation**: The methanol in aspartame is toxic. **Not supported**. While methanol is a by-product of aspartame digestion, it is not foreign to the human diet. The pectin in many common foods including fruits and vegetables and their juices contains low levels of methanol and substances that are metabolized to methanol. A cup of tomato juice would provide about six times more methanol than a cup of aspartame-containing soft drink. Dietary methanol, whether it comes from aspartame or common foods, is present at levels too low to cause any health problems. It does not accumulate in the body but is metabolized through normal metabolic pathways to form-

aldehyde, then to **formic acid** and finally to **water and carbon dioxide**. "

All this sounds fine, except one thing. It **presumes** that your metabolism is healthy enough to convert (neutralize) quickly the methanol into harmless water and Carbon Dioxide. I have heard so many times obese people to say: "Whatever I eat sticks to my body". Their metabolism cannot manage even with the simple conversions of carbohydrates and fats into energy.

Then we can reasonably question how successfully, and especially **quickly,** their bodies can get rid of the **formic acid**. What's the problem with it? It is simply the strongest organic acid in the world! If a concentrated drop falls on your leg, it will burn a whole in the tissue and then in the bone. Fire ants secrete exactly formic acid, which makes them very dangerous for human beings.

To sum up, what I believe is the **safest** approach to aspartame:

1. Pregnant and lactating women should **never** take pure non-food sources of phenylalanine such as **aspartame, sweeteners, soft drinks, chewing gums and sweetened supplements**. At the same time, they should take moderate quantities of foods, providing the essential amino acid- phenylalanine. They must avoid also **chocolate**, which contains significant amount of this amino acid, **caffeine** and **teobromin**. These 2 substances may further affect the brain and the nervous system of their babies (see **Caffeine** later on in The Directory)
2. Since you are not a baby, the important thing is how healthy you consider your metabolism. If it is good then you can safely eat or drink in **moderate quantities** anything, which contains aspartame. Usually its

quantity is very small. Furthermore, as Health Canada says with the approval of other sweeteners, which are also challenged for side effects, aspartame's presence in products will drop.

3. If you are overweight, I strongly recommend that you **avoid** the richest sources of aspartame- soft drinks and sweeteners. The problem is that **optimum acidity, metabolism and hydration** surely lack in your body. These 3 key, yet neglected points are the reason why "one-size-fits-all" diets, weight lose programs and fitness efforts are in the best case **useless** for substantial and permanent weight optimization.

That's why I called my next book "Your Scientific Diet®" because it keeps you focused on these **3 scientific and crucial points**. If they are **not** optimum, you can only suffer in order to reduce your weight without any significant and long term results. Furthermore, you will be more vulnerable to potential side effects from common substances such as aspartame.

I am amazed at the popular crash diets, which millions of people especially in the USA follow **blindly**. The result from them is a shocking increase in obesity (61% above 16) as well as a **boom of diabetes** and heart attacks. The major problem is that these "one-size-fits-all" diets and programs do not take into consideration your **unique:**

genetic inheritance
speed of metabolism
current health condition

as well as **your**:

-   dominating nervous system- Para/sympathetic
-   drugs and supplements you take

- internal optimum pH
- local climate
- gender

All these are 8 very important factors, which directly or indirectly affect the way your body processes all nutrients, vitamins, minerals, amino acids and substances. That's why unless you follow at least a partially customized overall program for your unique body, intoxication and overweight will be problematic for you.

The Controversial Amino Acid-Phenylalanine

Why is it important

L-phenylalanine is an **essential** amino acid, which means that your body cannot produce it on its own. It plays a major role as a building block of the proteins in the body and is the precursor of L-tyrosine.

Where is it found naturally

It occurs mainly in foods rich in proteins, such as eggs, milk and wheat.

Who needs it and what are the symptoms of deficiency

The chances to be deficient are very little. A healthy diet, which contains protein-rich foods, provides a sufficient amount of it. As a whole, it is not an amino acid you should think about.

Are there any side effects

<u>If you take high doses for more than few weeks-</u> **YES!** As you have learnt from the section for Aspartame, high blood concentration of phenylalanine can negatively affect your brain and its normal functioning. That's why FDA recommends that you **avoid** taking supplements, which contain high doses of <u>manufactured</u> L-phenylalanine. You should get enough from your food.

In case that you have a reasonable need, use **whey or soy protein** as a supplement. They naturally contain all essential amino acids, including phenylalanine. The digestion of food takes time and the food-bond amino acids enter gradually in the blood stream. Moreover, you can hardly take high dose of any amino acid from food. Thus the risk from potentially dangerous "high concentration" is eliminated.

Important note: You can find formulas, which aim at the morning sleepiness. However, they contain <u>huge doses</u> of caffeine, phenylalanine, teobromin, Guarana and other stimulants, which can really "blast" your mood and "lift you up" so high, that **you can drop dead!** You must avoid them. If you have such problems, a tablet with <u>L-tyrosine</u> will work wonders for you.

Tryptophan- the Other Controversial Amino Acid

Why is it important

Tryptophan is also one of the 8 essential amino acids. It is the precursor of 5-HTP and Serotonin.

Where is it found naturally

Foods particularly rich in this amino acid are oats, bananas, cottage cheese, dried dates, fish, meat, milk, peanuts and turkey.

Are there any side effects

In 1980, the FDA found a large batch of Japanese tryptophan with **impurities** left from the fermentation and/or filtration process. They caused symptoms of EMS (eosinophilia-myalgia syndrome). In 1989, cases of an unusual syndrome were observed. It was associated with strong muscular and abdominal pain, weakness, exertional dyspnea, mouth ulcers, skin rash and associated greatly elevated levels of particular white blood cells. The patients had taken over a period of 3 weeks to 1.5 years tryptophan in doses of 1.2 to 2.4 g/day as a treatment of insomnia. This disorder was termed "tryptophan-induced eosinophilia-myalgia.

By February 1990, the Centers for Disease Control (CDC) had been notified of 1,269 similar cases, associated with taking supplemental tryptophan. On the FDA's web site, there is a warning for these additional batches with impurities similar to the Japanese batches of tryptophan in 1980. As a result, FDA has banned the sales of manufactured tryptophan. That's why you have to **be extremely careful**!

I personally will never use <u>manufactured</u> tryptophan. Instead, I eat enough from the foods, which provide this essential amino acid. As an additional source, I take <u>whey protein</u> daily. It contains **natural** phenylalanine and tryptophan, which are considered safe. Actually, you can hardly get enough tryptophan from natural sources to experience any adverse reactions.

5-HTP (5-Hydroxy-tryptophan)

Why is it important

5-HTP (5-Hydroxy-tryptophan) is a metabolite of the amino acid tryptophan. It **directly converts** in the brain into a chemical called **Serotonin**. As you already know, it is an important inhibitory neurotransmitter related to **Dopamine**. Serotonin is known as 5-HT or 5-hydroxy-tryptamine. It is found in several places in the body, particularly the brain, gastrointestinal system and blood cells. There is a direct relation between the stressful way of life and the low levels of Serotonin in the brain. Unfortunately, this causes many health problems.

Where is it found naturally

The richest natural sources are protein-rich foods such as milk, cheese, turkey, fish, bananas, peanuts and dried dates.

What are its functions

As one of the three major neurotransmitters, Serotonin has many important functions in the human body. For example, it is secreted in response to mood or emotional swings. However, its major function is to placate and **calm you down**. People often experience a feeling of satisfaction when the levels of this fantastic neurotransmitter are the way they should be. Serotonin has 4 main areas of impact:

mood
behavior
appetite
sleep

Who needs it and what are the symptoms of deficiency

Nowadays, there are more and more people with the so called "low serotonin syndrome". It develops mainly as a result of <u>serious daily stress</u>. The importance of sufficient levels of **tryptophan - 5-HTP - Serotonin** for normal behaviour, appetite, mood and sleep has been well-known for years.

So far, many clinical studies have been conducted to evaluate the potential of 5-HTP to cure several common and serious health problems. The results range from **significant to impressive**. Here are 16 health issues, which are connected with deficiency of this neurotransmitter. They start with the mostly reduced problem from 5-HTP:

- migraine headaches
- tension headaches
- chronic daily headaches
- depression
- anxiety
- insomnia
- narcolepsy
- sleep apnea
- post menstrual syndrome
- obsessive/compulsive behavior
- obesity due to emotional eating
- vague muscle aches
- exhaustion
- carbohydrates craving
- bulimia
- fibromyalgia

5-HTP has been used to prevent headaches for a long time. People who often suffer from such problems **al-**

ways have low levels of Serotonin. That's why the results from several studies using 5-HTP for migraine and tension headaches show very good results!

Research also shows that 5-HTP is a very effective **antidepressant**. For example, there was an interesting study conducted with 99 patients. None of them responded to normal antidepressants. They were given an average of 200 mg/day of 5-HTP. **43** of the 99 participants reported a **complete recovery** while 8 others reported a significant improvement.

Is there a recommended dose and any side effects

You have already learnt about the health hazards of supplemental **manufactured** tryptophan. Though related to it, 5-HTP is a different substance. I am very glad that after the incidents with the Japanese batches other ways for their manufacturing have been sought. Nowadays, the good laboratories have stopped using fermentation-filtration process, which mainly caused the problems with EMS.

Instead, they extract 5-HTP from the seeds of Griffonia Simplicifolia plant. As a result, the FDA has received much fewer reports for health problems caused by it. Although it is **safer than tryptophan,** there is still a small possibility for the occurrence of EMS. There have been some cases of EMS-like symptoms after 5-HTP supplementation. It is difficult to say whether there is a direct correlation, because EMS can occur on its own.

There aren't clear evidences for the safety of a long-term use of 5-HTP. That's why the best approach is to take the minimum effective dosage and stop the day when your problem is eliminated or under control. Then continue with natural sources of the precursor L-tryptophan.

Where can I get it

5-HTP is available in most online supplemental stores and is very affordable, though you should **not** take and use more than one bottle. I have searched for supplements at Google's product search engine www.froogle. com. Here is the best keyword phrase:

pharmaceutical grade 5-HTP Griffonia

Important note: the most well-known and common description of certain supplements on the web sites is "pharmaceutical grade". However, you can use "**pure**" or "**USP**" instead. In this way, you can find several more companies and supplements, which are also top quality and contain minor amounts of impurities.

The Amino Acid- L-Arginine

Why is it important

L-Arginine is a naturally-occurring, semi-essential amino acid. It participates in many important biochemical reactions associated with the normal physiology of your body. Since it is difficult to make it on its own, it is important to consume foods that are rich in Arginine.

Where is it found naturally

There are high concentrations of it in nuts and seeds like peanuts, almonds and raisins. Arginine is present in various amounts in all protein-rich foods. Dairy products, meat, poultry and fish are especially good sources.

What are its functions

Arginine is necessary for the execution of many physiological processes such as

- hormone secretion of insulin and HGH
- removal of toxic waste products from the body
- immune system defense
- blood vasodilatation

The stimulation of hormonal release is mainly related with the production of HGH (Human Growth Hormone) from the pituitary gland. Mainly its metabolite **Arginine Pyroglutamate** has the ability to pass the brain-blood barrier more easily.

What is its scientific importance

Arginine is the precursor of NO (Nitric Oxide), which is responsible for the vasodilatation. That's why Arginine is often used for the treatment of conditions such as

- Angina pectoris
- Hypertension
- Erectile dysfunction
- Coronary artery diseases
- Sterility associated with Oligospermia
- Female infertility
- Atherosclerosis
- Hypercholesterolemia (high cholesterol)
- Nephrosclerosis associated with diabetes mellitus

Recently, dietary supplements containing Arginine have become popular due to Arginine's ability to

- produce Nitric Oxide
- scavenge free radicals

- promote erection
- release Growth Hormone
- remove bad cholesterol
- enhance fat metabolism
- increase muscles' fuel creatine as its indirect precursor

Clinical studies show that it also helps with the regulation of salt levels in the body. It also plays an important role in the protein synthesis and muscle growth. This makes it popular among athletes who want to increase their lean muscle mass.

It strengthens the immune system and stimulates the size and activity of the Thymus gland, which is responsible for the production of the immune system's T-cells. This makes it an excellent option for HIV patients and for anyone recovering from an injury.

It is often linked to sexual stimuli with the idea that it may lengthen and improve orgasms. It is present in the seminal fluid and is often used in studies to improve the male sexual health.

It also improves the health of the liver, skin and the connective tissues. Mostly Arginine facilitates the gain of lean muscle mass while limiting fat storage. This is due to its ability to keep fat circulating and burning in the body. It is a key ingredient in many weight control formulas.

Who needs it and what are the symptoms of deficiency

People who mainly need Arginine are children, athletes, elderly and obese people. In adults, Arginine is considered a non-essential amino acid. For children, by contrast, Arginine is essential for the defense and development of the adolescent immune system.

People suffering from an injury can greatly benefit from it. The demand for Arginine in the body increases during times of injury and restoration. Men suffering from erectile dysfunction or poor blood circulation benefit from using Arginine because of its vasodilating properties. This amino acid increases the diameter of the blood vessels. In this way, it helps greater blood flow to reach the genital area.

Clinical studies show that men with a low sperm count have had an increase in the number of spermatozoids after supplementation with L-Arginine. If you want to increase your ejaculation volume, make sure that you have high intake of this amino acid.

Supplementing with Arginine may boost the immune system and help reverse conditions, such as hypertension. In combination with **Niacin** (Vitamin B3), it fights the accumulation of bad cholesterol in the body.

As a result from Arginine's ability to:

- increase Growth Hormone levels
- encourage lipid (fat) oxidization
- lower blood pressure
- decrease arterial plaque

it is beneficial for obese people.

Is there a recommended dose

Daily consumption of 1-2 grams is usually appropriate for a healthy individual. You can consult with your physician to determine the optimal intake of Arginine to improve your performance or recover from a serious trauma.

Research has shown that daily consumption of 1-2 grams of L-Arginine combined with weight training has led to decrease in body fat within five weeks.

Are there any side effects

We do not know about direct side effects. If you have an existing heart, liver or kidney disease or you are sensitive to herpes viruses, consult with your physician before taking supplements containing Arginine. At this time, there are no well-known drug interactions.

As with any product containing amino acid, there is a possibility for overdose. Taking too much Arginine can lead to diarrhea, weakness and nausea. Clear dosing guidelines have not yet been established. That's why you can take a small dosage for one week and note the benefits. You can gradually increase the dosage until the benefits are maximized. However, it is always better to follow the directions as prescribed on the label.

Where can I get it

Several brand manufacturers provide **pharmaceutical grade Arginine**. Check in your local pharmacy or favourite online store.

The Erectile Neurotransmitter Nitric Oxide

Why is it important

Nitric Oxide is a free form gas. It is a key molecule, manufactured by the body, which causes vasodilatation (expansion of the internal diameter of blood vessels). This leads to increased blood flow, Oxygen transport, delivery of nutrients and reduction in blood pressure. Its production requires the break down of Arginine from enzymes. Nitric Oxide occurs when the amino acid L-Arginine converts into L-Citruline.

What are its functions

The best short profile of NO I have read is from the Royal Society and Association of British Science Writers. Here is a brief excerpt:

"Summary research papers continue to flood the scientific journals and insights into the biological activity and potential clinical uses of Nitric Oxide (NO): a gas controlling a seemingly limitless range of functions in the body. Each revelation adds to Nitric Oxide's already lengthy resume in controlling the circulation of the blood, regulating activities of the brain, lungs, liver, kidneys, stomach and other organs.

The molecule governs blood pressure through a recently recognized process that contradicts textbook wisdom. It causes penile erection by dilating blood vessels and controls the action of almost every orifice from swallowing to defecation. The immune system uses Nitric Oxide in fighting viral, bacterial and parasitic infections, and tumors. Nitric Oxide transmits messages between nerve cells and is associated with the process of learning, memory, sleeping, feeling pain, and probably depression. It is a mediator in inflammation and rheumatism."

Nitric Oxide also has an impact on the endocrine system by affecting the release of the HGH and Adrenaline.

Who needs it

Everyone needs plenty of Nitric Oxide to carry out key physiological processes within their body. From a penis enlargement perspective, NO donating supplements are used to increase the blood flow to your genital area. Men suffering from erectile dysfunction will also find supplementing with Nitric Oxide helpful.

What are the symptoms of deficiency

Signs of deficiency include inability to achieve and sustain erections, physical weakness and extreme fatigue. Most "Nitric Oxide" supplements contain the amino acid compound **Arginine-alpha-keto-glutarate** (AAKG) and/ or **Arginine-keto-isocaproate**. Both of them can boost in short term the levels of Nitric Oxide. You can expect increased strength and improved stamina.

The most valued amino acids for increased levels of NO are L- Citruline and L- Ornithine. On one hand, L-Citruline is an amino acid that is an **extremely powerful** NO donor. This little known amino acid has a significant role in the production of NO. This is due to its unique ability to recycle itself continuously into NO. This continuous process promotes increased and relatively sustained levels of NO in the blood. On the other hand, L- Ornithine converts into L-Arginine, which produces NO. These 3 key amino acids are very helpful to achieve a greater amount of Nitric Oxide in the blood.

Very important in the chemical chain of conversions is the enzyme Nicotinamide Adenine Dinucleotide (NAD). In the ingredients of multivitamin formulas, you can find its precursor "Nicotinamide" or "Vitamin B3". It is an essential NO enzyme that has a vital role in the conversion of AAKG into NO. Without this enzyme, NO conversion is minimized to small levels. Make sure that your multivitamin formula provides sufficient amounts of it for maximum support to optimum production of NO in your body.

Is there a recommended dose and any side effects

As with any product, containing amino acid, overdose is a possibility. Taking too much Arginine can lead to diarrhea, weakness and nausea. It is best to follow the instruction on the label. Many protein powders are fortified with amino acids, including Arginine. Having this in mind, pay particular attention to how much Arginine you are ingesting from all supplements. There are no well-known side effects.

Where can I get it

If you have to boost the NO levels in your body, you can search for supplements at www.froogle.com using any of the following keyword phrases:

pharmaceutical grade arginine-alpha ketoglutarate
pharmaceutical grade arginine ketoisocaproate
pharmaceutical grade ornithin

Choline (Acetylcholine's precursor)

Why is it important

Choline acts as a cell-signalling molecule, as a precursor of Acetylcholine and adds structural integrity to the cells' membranes.

What are its functions

The main responsibility of Choline is the production of the neurotransmitter of the Parasympathetic Nervous

System - **Acetylcholine**. It is released in the brain and in neuromuscular junctions. It is responsible for numerous and vital physiological processes.

Studies show that the concentration of choline in the blood of athletes can drop by up to **40%** during trainings. These reductions automatically lead to a reduction in acetylcholine synthesis. This negatively affects your focus and (sexual) performance. Choline supplementation can replenish these reduced blood choline concentrations.

Due to its effects on acetylcholine levels in the brain, choline supplementation can enhance memory capacity in healthy people. Furthermore, choline, together with substances that prolong the effects of Acetylcholine at the neuromuscular junction, may improve neuromuscular transmission. **Supplemental lecithin** is very common and affordable. It provides phosphatidylcholine, which directly increases the available choline in the body. However, if you want a superior donor, it is definitely **cytidine-5-diphosphocholine**. What is unique for this little known substance is that it easily passes the brain-blood barrier and very quickly converts into Acetylcholine.

Where is it found naturally

Choline, especially from lecithin, is a basic dietary substance found in many protein and fat-containing foods such as eggs, meats, soybeans, peanuts, etc.

Is there a recommended dose

A healthy diet and the recommended from FDA adequate intake of 550 mg/day is a good foundation for most men. The FDA's upper tolerable limit is the looping 3.5 g per day. However, for periods of intensive fitness or sexual activity, it is necessary to take at least 1 g of choline per day.

Lecithin may act synergistically with the sugar cane or rice derived supplement **policosanol**, which is also helpful for cholesterol problems. It increases the action of acetylcholine at the neuromuscular junction. However, be careful, because up to certain degree and dosage of both substances your muscle tone will get better. But after that, your muscles will start getting **stiff**. Fitness lovers and elderly people who need more Acetylcholine may try to find out their optimum dosage between 1 g and the FDA's upper limit of 3.5 g.

Are there any side effects

According to the FDA, if the intake of choline is higher than 3.5 g/day, the adverse effects can be "hypotension (low blood pressure), with sweating, diarrhea and fishy body odor."

Where can I get it

When performing a search, use the keyword phrases:

pharmaceutical grade cytidine-5-diphosphocholine
pharmaceutical grade lecithin B5 bha
pharmaceutical grade choline bitartrate
pharmaceutical grade choline
policosanol

L-Tyrosine (Dopamine's precursor)

Why is it important

L-tyrosine is a nonessential organic amino acid, which takes part in the building-up of lean muscle mass. It is the precursor of the neurotransmitter Dopamine and the stress hormone Epinephrine (Adrenalin).

Where is it found naturally

The body can make L-tyrosine from the essential amino acid phenylalanine. Foods, rich in L-tyrosine, include animal meat, wheat products, oatmeal and seafood.

What are its functions

L-tyrosine has the ability to offset physical and mental fatigue as a precursor of Dopamine. That's why it can help men to avoid over-training and a drop in their sexual performance or capabilities. Supplementing with L-tyrosine may heighten mental alertness, increase feelings of well being and ease depression.

Who needs it and what are the symptoms of deficiency

The people with greatest need for it are athletes, elderly and obese people. If you are regularly involved in high intensity or stressful activities (training, work, sex), make sure that you supply **a lot of** L-tyrosine. This amino acid is also necessary for the production of the dark pigment Melanin, which protects your skin from the ultraviolet light of the sun. That's why if you want to sunbathe, take a moment to evaluate the level of preparation of your body. If your goal is to achieve nice tan, abundance of L-tyrosine is essential.

L-Tyrosine is helpful for people with:

- anxiety
- premature ejaculation
- narcolepsy
- low sex drive

- depression
- allergies
- chronic fatigue
- headaches

People having these problems usually have low blood levels of this amino acid. That's why supplementing is <u>highly recommended</u>.

L-tyrosine converts also into the thyroid hormone thyroxin. It has a **direct impact on the basal metabolic rate**. That's why L-tyrosine may prove effective for weight loss. This amino acid is appropriate for supporting the immune system against AIDS or hepatitis. Furthermore, it is helpful for retaining skeletal muscles and anabolic environment. This is important to increase your lean muscle mass and burn fat.

Is there a recommended dose and any side effects

As with any product, containing amino acid, overdose is a possibility. There are no clear dosing guidelines, so it is better to follow the instructions on the label. Many protein powders are fortified with amino acids, including tyrosine. Having this in mind, pay attention to how much you are ingesting from all supplements. There are **no** well-known side effects.

Where can I get it

Many brand names manufacture supplemental L-Tyrosine. Here are the best keyword phrases:

- pharmaceutical grade tyrosine
- pure tyrosine
- USP tyrosine

Little Known Facts about (Soy) Protein

Why is it important

Soy protein is one of the few, which rank high in the Protein Digestibility Corrected Amino Acid Score (PDCAAS). In general, it is nearly free of fat, cholesterol and lactose. That's why it is appropriate for lactose-intolerant people. Furthermore, it is appropriate as a meat and flour substitute and a very affordable ingredient for protein shakes. Soy protein is derived exclusively from soybeans. That's why it is an excellent and natural ingredient for the production of high protein foods, which contain extremely low fat. This is traditionally desired by fitness lovers!

What are its functions

Soy protein provides **all amino acids** as well as **saponins**, **phytosterols** and **isoflavones**. Saponins improve the function of the immune system and are used with a certain success in cancer treatment studies. Furthermore, they react with the cholesterol to reduce its absorption in the body through the small intestine. Phytosterols have a similar effect. Soy protein supplies non-animal protein in the diet. This makes it especially appropriate for vegetarians and people with problematic levels of cholesterol.

The **isoflavones** in soy are nature's best protection against the accumulation of DHT and successfully detoxify it from the male body. Furthermore, the specific forms **genistein** and **daidzein** have anabolic effect and are very powerful antioxidants. Studies show that they may reduce the risk of hormone-dependent cancer of prostate and other cancers as well.

Are there any side effects

Soy protein is generally safe except for people who are allergic to it. Since it contains all amino acids, consult with your physician if you are on any prescription drugs. Soy contains phytic acid, which can decrease the absorption of calcium. That's why do **not** go overboard with the amounts you take or increase the intake of this mineral. If you train a lot then **whey protein** is definitely preferable for greater intake. It is a little bit more expensive, although it provides outstanding value and quality in return for your money.

"Ecstasy" versus Top Chinese Herbs for Great Vigor, Increased Fertility and Steel Erections

When it comes to Chinese herbs, I can hardly remain objective. Since the day I experienced the instant amazing effect of **Schizandra and Lycium drops,** I was deeply impressed and intrigued by the Traditional Chinese Herbology. Now, I am with the confidence of a semi-expert in this field.

A particular expert stands out from the rest. When you combine his in-depth knowledge of hundreds of sophisticated Chinese herbs with his commitment to superior quality, the result is unsurpassed herbal products. I will not reveal his name or company because it is not necessary. If you search a little bit in the Internet, you will immediately find him. There are thousands of sites, which try to sell you their herbal products right away. On the contrary, you can spend 1 week on his 3 sites reading **hundreds of pages** with first class information provided for free. I wish there were more people like him.

When it comes to Chinese herbs, his informative sites and products are simply the best in the world. The rest are very far behind. He has won me as a loyal customer and I simply cannot imagine my life without the top Chinese herbs. In fact, I love them so much that around 50% of the money I spend annually on supplements is exactly for top Chinese herbs. I guarantee you that you have to try **just once** for example Schizandra and Lycium drops or Siberian Ginseng drops. Then you will be blown away by their instant **almost magical** effect on your body and mind.

It is amazing how much money people spend on harmful, addictive and expensive products like cigarettes, alcohol and illegal drugs. Furthermore, the quantity is enough for only a couple of days. On the contrary, a bottle of Schizandra and Lycium drops for example costs about **$22** and lasts **4-6 months**. Since it is a "super-extract", a few drops in the morning are more than enough to work their magic on you. No cigarettes, alcohol, illegal drugs or something else will ever give you even **1/50** of the bliss and harmony, which several drops of **any Top 10 Chinese herbs can**!

You should definitely consider at least <u>Schizandra</u>. You can spend more than 1 hour reading everything that expert has written about it on his sites. However, you have to **experience it** for yourself why it is referred to as the <u>master Chinese herb</u> and stands right next to **Ginseng**.

Talking about almost "magical" substances, have you ever used 3,4-methyl-deoxy-meta-1-phenyl-2-propyl-amine, which is also known as **Ecstasy**? If you take it or have thought about this, you had better **stop**. Its neurophysiologic effect is to release the whole Serotonin stored in your body, causing a huge confidence and power boosting. At the same time, it blocks the mechanism for its restoring.

When such a huge dose of Serotonin rushes in your body you may feel like a Superman for a few hours. However, once it converts into Melatonin, you will feel like a **doormat for up to 3 days**! The bigger problem is that most people do **not** know how to replenish the amount of Serotonin in their body. That's why they end up with a severe deficiency very quickly!

However, the greatest argument against Ecstasy is that after taking several pills, **deformations** of the membranes in the brain will occur, which act as doors of the stores for Serotonin. That's why repeated use leads to very serious psychological problems. Unfortunately, once these executive membranes are severely deformed, the modern medicine can do nothing.

Furthermore, the resulting constant leaking of Serotonin will trigger constant conversion into Melatonin and increased production of Adrenaline from Dopamine. It is really a nasty future (constant drowsiness and irrational anxiety or depression) for only several hours of **illusive** power and happiness.

With the money for 2-3 pills Ecstasy, you can enjoy the outstanding benefits of Schizandra and Lycium drops for a **whole year** without any addiction, side effects and illusive bliss and energy on a daily basis. The other similar pills, such as amphetamines, ketamines, LSD, etc., slowly but steadily drag to the bottom everyone who has had the ignorance or stupidity to start taking them.

I will not even discuss hard drugs such as heroin and cocaine. With **90% certainty** to finish your life worse than a dog in an uninhabited area or building is only an option for people who want to commit suicide.

If you consider the ratio **pleasure:side effects:price per milligram,** the top Chinese herbs are <u>far ahead</u> of any illegal drug. Sometimes at teen groups and chats, I reach the point to read: "You, daddy, doesn't know what is to feel and live at the max!" My standard reply is: "In fact, **you** have no clue what **really** is to feel and live at the maximum 365 days per year." Then I share step-by-step only few of the things that you keep on learning from this book and they are amazed from the pleasure and results. I can confidently say that I know the ins and outs of every single common and little known substance out there, which can directly or indirectly help you to feel and live at the **maximum 365 days per year**.

Everything, which is **not** in this book or does **not** have positive comments, is definitely **NOT** worth your attention, time and money. Only people like me can take illegal drugs because we know their "positive" and side effects. However, we will **never do** it because they all are crap and everyone who gets involved with them sooner or later becomes **good for nothing**. This is sad but fact, which you can check at the web sites of anonymous drug addicts, alcoholics, etc.

I was amazed to learn that an average British family spends annually £800 **($1,460)** only for **alcohol. No** wonder that in the UK there are more than **2 million impotent men** because it suppresses the testosterone levels. If they spent this money to live really at the maximum instead of destroying their health and lives, the situation would be very different. It is your life and I do hope that you will live it at its optimum just like me **without becoming a slave** of pills, injections, alcohol, cigarettes or something else.

Here I have provided 3 lists mainly with Chinese herbs starting with the most effective or potent one. The first list is for those men who want to increase their fertility. Once again, I want to remind the crucial importance of

- drinking plenty of water
- taking enough L-Arginine
- making regularly the VIP Genital Massage
- taking Evening Primrose or Borage/Starflower oil

Polygonum Multiflorum Root- an exceptional herb, which can significantly increase your sperm count. This is the most potent Chinese herb for this purpose and one of the premium ones. It is also superior for anti-aging purposes. This is the leading herb in one of the most popular Chinese formulas: **Shou Wu Formulation**. When it is time to fertilize your lady I strongly recommend that you start using it 4-5 months in advance. I agree that this is a long period. However, it takes **3 months** for a spermatozoid to mature in your testicles and be able to go out and give the beginning of a new life. That's why if you start using it today, the peak result will be noticeable after 3 months.

Epimedium Sagittatum (Horny Goat Weed) is currently the best selling natural anti depressant. However, it also increases the sperm production and acts just like Viagra/Cialis without their side effects. If you are already very sexually active, **avoid** using it because it will drive you wild. Also, it is not appropriate for long-term use because of its drying effect as well as for people who suffer from dryness. The active substance in this herb is **icariin**. This is a very, very interesting substance, which has both a positive and not that positive side.

On one hand, it interferes with the break down of cGMP from PDE-5 just like Viagra and Cialis. Thus, it helps men to keep their erection longer. Compared to the 2 drugs it is slower and shorter acting, which I consider also benefits. In general, I am **against** the use of high doses of strong inhibitors such as Serotonin, GABA, HGH Secretagogue, Icariin and Viagra type of drugs! There are regulatory mechanisms in our bodies which were established million of years ago. It is in our best interest to respect them and do **not** seriously interfere in their functions.

Can icariin cure erectile dysfunction? There was a very thorough study conducted in China aiming to answer this question and the results were published in "Asian J Androl 2003 Mar; 5: 15-18". You can type this reference exactly as I have written it at Google and read the article online. The result is **positive**. Icariin, in a dose-dependent way, can inhibit the release of PDE-5 enzyme just like Viagra and Cialis, thus prolonging the erection. When you compare the lowest prices of one-month supply from icariin and Viagra, the ratio is **1:7**. For Cialis it is **1:15**. The good side is definitely very impressive.

I want to warn you for one more thing in addition to undesirable regular, long-term use. Icariin inhibits the enzyme called **Acetylcholinesterase** (AChE) in your body. Its function is to break the acetylcholine into acetic acid and choline. You may consider it actually bad but it is **not** so.

When a nerve signal has to pass from one nerve cell to another, Acetylcholine is synthesized at the place of their junction, which allows the transition. Once the signal passes, AChE breaks the acetylcholine and in this way **stops the signal**. When another signal comes, everything starts again. Your nervous system functions in this way. If it is an enjoyable signal and a substance, such as icariin, blocks AChE, this will prolong the nervous signal (pleasure). This is surely good.

However, when we have the case with nerve and muscle cells, the situation is exactly the opposite. Let's say that you have penetrated in your lady and want to pull out. The AChE has to break the Acetylcholine, thus stopping the command "push", so that the new command "pull out" can be executed. If because of icariin AChE can **not** do its job then becomes a **communication mess**. You will definitely feel it as some uncomfortable and gradually **stiff feeling** in your working muscles. Is the inhibiting of AChE a big deal? Yes, and the proof is that venomous snakes kill people exactly by severely inhibiting AChE. For your nervous system, icariin will act just like diluted snake's poison.

But is it possible to take small enough but effective dose to support your erection without interfering too much with the AChE's functions? This depends on the man. However, you have complete information how to eliminate an erectile dysfunction (impotence) if you have such issue. That's why icariin has little to offer to perfectly sexually healthy men.

I would say that just like GABA, it can be an "Ace in the slave" when the duration of sex is very important. However, **NEVER** take GABA and icariin in a short time frame because both of them have inhibitory effect on the functions of Acetylcholine. If you want to evaluate for yourself the effect of Horny Goat Weed, here is the best keyword, which you may use at www.froogle.com

standardized extract 10% icariin

Male Silk Moth drops accelerate the growth of the sperm. In addition, it is one of the strongest male sexual stimulants. It can drive you sexually crazy for a female. It is like a premium herb, which is not very appropriate for everyday use because of its mild androgenic effect on the testicles. In addition, it is more expensive than the others, which makes it appropriate for special occasions and "Ace in the slave".

Cuscuta seed nourishes the sperm. If you have a temperature or fever, avoid taking it. This excellent herb is traditionally combined with **Cnidium seed** because they enhance each other.

Astragalus root is the only Chinese herb, which can improve the <u>mobility of spermatozoids</u>. You should not use it during flu.

Bulgarian Tribulus terrestris- it stimulates spermatogenesis- the number and quality of produced spermatozoids. In addition, it has clinically proven testosterone-boosting effect, which makes it very good for problems with the hardness of your erection. Of course, your liver has to provide enough 5-alpha-reductaze. Otherwise, there will be **no** conversion into DHT.

Shatawari, although not a Chinese herb, may increase sperm count and at the same time decrease spermatorrhea.

Combination of Folic acid and Zinc has improved the overall sperm count in subfertile men by **74%**. This is the impressive result from a research conducted by the University Medical Center in Nijmegen, The Netherlands and Tygerberg Hospital and University of Stellenbosch in South Africa. It proves that a regular intake of great multivitamin/mineral formula will protect you to a great extend from having such health issues.

Flax seed oil, which has become very popular, also benefits the sperm production.

The following <u>second list</u> provides several Chinese herbs, which are superior for **penis enlargement assistance**. I want to underline once again that it takes much more than greater blood volume and pressure in the penis to achieve permanent and significant enlargement. Here is a list with the vital substances and Chinese herbs, which can direct great amounts of blood towards your penis and genitals.

Mineral Water- this is the first and foremost component of any successful increasing in the blood volume and pressure in an erected penis. It is necessary to drink **minimum 2.5 liters** of preferably mineral water with low mineralization.

Arginine/Ornithine/Citruline- as you already know, they are extremely important for the production of the erectile neurotransmitter NO (Nitric Oxide). It manages the maximum filling of your penis with blood.

Cistanche is a little known herb, which has been used in China for centuries for harder erections and gradual penis enlargement. From all the herbs in the world, it is the **most effective** for increasing the blood flow to the penis. However, you will not find it in any of the popular formulas for penis enlargement. They contain herbs like Ginkgo Biloba, which have general vasodilating effect. That's why for enlargement purposes they have to be combined with herb(s) such as Cistanche.

Astragalus root is also very effective for increasing the blood flow to the lower part of the body, and in particular to the genitals. In addition, it increases the sexual energy.

Dong Qui is the premium herb, which increases the production of blood in the body.

Ginkgo Biloba is one of the most widely used herbs in the world today. The active ingredients in it are quercetin and proanthocyanidins, which have extremely powerful antioxidant properties. You can find these 2 great substances in advanced multi formulas. Furthermore, this herb significantly improves the supply of Oxygen to the brain and improves the blood circulation in the body. It can act synergistically with the herbs above.

The third list presents the premium or top Chinese herbs, which are considered **adaptogens** or **moderators**. They have the unique abilities to work effectively in opposite directions depending on your body's needs. The following are the most powerful, all-purpose herbs, which have been used in the Chinese Herbology for 2000-3000 years.

Panax Ginseng- this is the most widely known and recognized herb in the world. Just like Schizandra, Ginseng benefits every single system and organ in the body. It has influence on both the Parasympathetic and Sympathetic nervous systems, which accounts for its **regulatory effect**. However, it is recommended to follow 3 weeks on and 1 week off schedule of intake. In this way, you will avoid too much depositing of some of the specific bioactive substances of Ginseng in your nervous system.

Schizandra and Lycium Drops- if you want to use only one product containing Chinese herbs, it should be this one. It will benefit every single organ and system in your body. In addition, it is believed that it has significant energizing and unblocking effect on the energy channels. Both herbs and especially Schizandra act on every level and on every major area in your body with impressive results. Also, it is one of the most widely used herbs for sexual energizing and ejaculation control.

Gynostemma (Southern Ginseng) - as one of the Top 3 in the Chinese Herbology, this is an extremely popular herb in Asia. Actually, it is a "cure-all" type of herb. It is the leading herb in my morning tea, which also contains Schizandra and Lycium. This is one of the premium health boosting and anti-aging combinations.

Reishi- it is considered one of the best herbs in the world. Its major area of influence is the strengthening of the immune system. In addition, it is excellent for anti-stress, inner balancing and wisdom developing.

Cordyceps and the 3 herbs below are specifically beneficial on physical and sexual level. Cordyceps has a deep nourishing and restorative effect on the body. In addition, it improves the respiratory function and the utilization of Oxygen, which is very important during exercises and sexual activity. A person who takes this herb will find it difficult to feel very tired and sick as a result from viruses and bacteria. It is a very strong immune-modulating and, when necessary, immune-strengthening herb.

Tibetan Rhodiola (Plateau Ginseng) - unbelievably, this herb is one of the major reasons for the impressive physical and spiritual achievements of the monks living in Tibet. It grows in extreme conditions very high in the Himalayas. That's why the only herb, which comes close to its overall effect on the body, is the Siberian Ginseng. Tibetan Rhodiola greatly increases the **resistance** to stress, weather conditions, fatigue, etc. However, in contrast with its Siberian equivalent, it greatly assists those who consume it to develop their wisdom and spiritual level. In addition to its effect on the body, Rhodiola deeply energizes and clears mental stress, helps you to stay focused and have balanced attitude towards life. It is a miracle that this rare herb is available outside of Tibet and China.

Siberian Ginseng Drops- just like the previous premium herbs in this list, the history of this herb dates back 2,000 years back. Although Shen Nong Ben Cao first classified it as a general class herb, later on another great master awarded it with "superior" status and I completely agree with him. This unimpressive at first sight bush grows only in the **harshest regions** of Siberia and Northern China. It has become one of the few legal stimulants permitted for use by the Olympic Committee. However, long before that, all Soviet astronauts and athletes had used it with outstanding results. I never go to the gym or make physical exercises at home without several drops of Siberian Ginseng and Tibetan Rhodiola plus 3 capsules of Cordyceps.

Few months ago, I was chatting with 19 years old teenager, who wrote to me:

- I will stop taking Ecstasy if you tell me something better, which does not have the side effects you wrote me about. (Well, this was an excellent chance to "outsell" the drug pills with **Siberian Ginseng, Rhodiola** and **Cordyceps**. After one week, he wrote me back.)
- You told me to use 3 capsules and 1 dropper but I liked the drops so much that I took a second dropper. Immediately, I felt fantastic and my mind was extremely clear. Then I went to a club, found a nice girl and later on, we had sex. I expected that this will be the weak point of these herbs because Ecstasy makes me last long. However, for the first time in my life, my dick was like made of steel and I lasted 40 minutes against 60 with Ecstasy. This was great and the best part was that on the next day, I was still feeling fantastic, with clear mind, full of positive energy and eager for action. Otherwise, I feel powerless and depressed for 2-3 days. These exotic herbs are really better, the

quantity is enough for few months and they are a lot cheaper than Ecstasy.
- Well, why didn't you tell me that you use Ecstasy as a sexual stimulant?
- Because you didn't ask me?
- (I like smart and funny guys) You still have **not** tried the very best Chinese herb for intensive sex!
- Really? Tell me about it!
- It is **Dendrobium**, the leading herb in a super extract with few other powerful herbs, which further increase its ultra fast and profound energizing of your entire sexual system.

Let's take a closer look at his words. Ecstasy does help to last long exactly because it deals with the management of **Serotonin** in the body. This is another confirmation for its crucial importance regarding sex and ejaculation control. However, the Siberian Ginseng and Cordyceps have a major impact on the sexual system, which results in its significant energizing and optimizing. When you combine this with Siberian Ginseng's superior optimizing effect on the central nervous system, it is logical that this combination can help men last longer.

Regarding the "steel" erection, it is mainly due to **Rhodiola**. It grows usually above 4,000 meters in the Himalayas, where Oxygen is very diluted. That's why it provides superior utilization of the Oxygen. This is especially important for the production of NO. The greater quantity of it is synthesized, the more your penis will be filled with blood. Siberian Ginseng, just like Rhodiola, also helps the body to utilize Oxygen to the maximum. However, the greatest effect comes from the combination of the 3 herbs.

Here is a list with the factors, which will give any sexually healthy man **steel erections**.

- minimum 2.5 liters of water daily
- at least 1 g of choline a day
- L-Arginine/Ornithin/Citruline
- Bulgarian Tribulus terrestris
- Cistanche, Dong Qui and Astragalus root
- Tibetan Rhodiola, Siberian Ginseng and Cordyceps

Dendrobium- it is the default herb, which people in Asia drink or take during their honeymoon. It is the best for the fast replenishing of used sexual energy and fluids. The #1 expert has formulated a super extract in which Dendrobium is the leading herb. I use few drops in the morning before sex in my tea and if I have a girlfriend in her tea as well. This super extract formulation is especially beneficial for women, because it supports the natural lubrication of the vagina and supports the production of blood and hormones. It is a deeply nourishing and energizing formula, which is a must for **honeymoon-grade** sexual activity.

One week after I wrote to that teenager for Dendrobium, he gave me the following feedback: "I will never even think for Ecstasy. Especially after using this new herb, I feel like Superman every single day and everyone around me is amazed at the change in my behaviour. My erections went from almost horizontal back to upright and my ejaculation volume almost tripled. My new girlfriend refuses to believe me that I have stopped taking Ecstasy. Today I will give her to try the herbs. Thanks a lot!"

One of the best sides of the Chinese herbs is their long term effect. Legal and illegal drugs have strong but short effect on the body plus serious side effects. On the contrary, the premium herbs I mentioned above may need few days to provide their peak effect and even if you stop taking them, you will still enjoy the benefits for a couple of days. This gentle to the body approach is definitely better than the drugs, especially when most of them have at least one serious side effect.

With 2,000-3,000 years safety record, the top Chinese herbs are the safest and most well known in the world. Many clinical studies confirm their healing and/or adaptogenic effects, which are already known from the traditional Chinese medicine.

Furthermore, when the #1 expert in this field provides a choice between dry powder in capsules and 10% alcohol-bond "super extracts", I always take the second one. The reason is that 1 drop is equal to 8 regular drops. That's why even 3 drops a day, which makes 24 regular drops, are more than enough to experience the full range of health benefits. In this way you still allow some accumulation of the active substances without overloading your body with them. It is also more affordable, because a single small bottle lasts for about 6 months.

I do hope that you will give them a chance to prove you that they are almost magical extracts, which can **dramatically improve** how you feel, look and behave. Also, they enter in the blood stream right from the mouth and you can feel their effect almost instantly. Usually I do **not** have hours to wait for a dry powder to be digested and to start utilizing once in the intestines.

The size of your pupils is one of the most reliable detectors if there is a strong psychoactive substance in your body. Illegal drugs such as Ecstasy, amphetamines, heroin, etc. push the Sympathetic nervous system to extremes. That's why the pupils always become like big dots. On the contrary, substances, which are beneficial for the body, act on and nurture the Parasympathetic nervous system. It energizes and relaxes the body. This is immediately obvious from the beautiful large pupils.

Caffeine

Caffeine affects the body mainly by stimulating the pro-duction of **Adrenalin**. It is a <u>strong diuretic</u>, although the similar substances teophilin and teobromin found in black tea and cacao have an even **stronger dehydrating effect**. Coffee stimulates very much the secretion of HCl (Hydrochloric Acid) in the stomach causing increased acidity. It also causes serious decalcification and weak-ening of the bones. That's why it is especially bad for women because in general they are in greater risk of **Osteoporosis**.

During an experiment with the bacteria *Escherichi coli,* high doses of caffeine have intensified the speed of the **destruction of DNA** and have caused considerable **mutations**! Such effect is not proven during a pregnancy, although it is known that caffeine restricts the blood flow towards the foetus, and this **slows down its development!** Now you know why women should **avoid** drinking coffee during pregnancy.

Regarding its affect on spermatozoids, I have found con-troversial studies. Some of them claim that it lowers their mobility, while others state exactly the opposite. I **always stand on the safe side** when it comes to substances. Take into consideration the **strong** diuretic, acidic, de-calcifying and Adrenalin-stress-premature ejaculation boosting properties of caffeine. Add and possible muta-genic/immobilizing effect on your spermatozoids. That's why I **completely avoid** it.

Caffeine, teophilin and teobromin have similar properties because they are part of one chemical group of substanc-es. The following are foods and drinks with considerable amount of caffeine, plus teophilin or teobromin for some of them. I have started with the most content-rich:

- Guarana (an ingredient in sex pills)
- coffee
- chocolate
- black tea
- Coca Cola
- Pepsi

Testosterone

What are its functions

Testosterone is the main steroid hormone in the male body. The major production comes from the Leydig cells of the testicles. Smaller amounts are produced in the adrenal glands. Testosterone has direct effect on the:

- strength, size and muscle definition
- body composition
- immune system
- mood and aggression
- cardiovascular system
- growth of the penis and testicles in your youth
- enlargement of the larynx for a deeper voice
- production of functional sperm
- stimulation of hair growth all over the body
- reductions in muscle glycogen breakdown during exercises
- regulation of prostate cancer (Nieschlag & Behre 1998)
- retention of sodium and water in the kidneys
- increased calcium retention and bone density
- increases in basal (resting) metabolic rate
- increases the total amount of red blood cells and blood volume
- increases skin thickness
- increases the libido

- increases muscle protein synthesis and mass
- increased activity of the sebaceous (sweat) glands

This list is **not** exhaustive because androgen hormones like testosterone participate in nearly every organ and cell of the body.

I want to give you some information in addition to Nieschlag and Behre's studies. **Enlargement** and development of **cancer of the prostate** has direct relation to the testosterone and DHT in your body. That's why isoflavones, and especially soy's genistein, are one of the most effective natural substances for fighting these conditions.

It is naïve to believe that these two very common problems will surely pass <u>you</u>. There were **220,900** new cases of prostate cancer in the USA only in 2003. I am sure that each of these men had done **NOTHING** to prevent this real danger, until their doctors told them: "You have cancer of the Prostate!" For 28,900 men in 2003, this meant a death sentence. **Prevention** is what every smart man should do.

Taking daily a top quality multi formula, which is recommended even by the conservative Journal of American Medical Association, is a good start. By top quality, I understand that a daily serving consists of at least 7 tablets, preferably more. This means more substances in total and higher amount from each one of them. Optimum health is achieved with optimum amounts, but without reaching the toxicity threshold for any of the components.

When I evaluate some multi-vitamin/mineral formula, the first thing I have in mind is the **prostate**! The reason is that only the most advanced formulas can completely protect and detoxify it. They cost extra several dollars, **but** also contain substances such as <u>boron</u>, which reduce the chances to end up one day with a potentially terminal disease. For me it is absolutely worth it. Here is the keyword phrase I use in www.google.com to track down the very best multi formulas money can buy.

polyphenols proanthocyanidins lycopene lutein hesperidin zinc boron choline

In order for a company to include such components in their formula, they have to have their own laboratory. This immediately means that they have the ambition to be a leader in the vitamin industry. Furthermore, they are controlled by government agencies for quality and standards.

Once I have few suggestions, the next step is to visit www.betterwhois.com. There I check since when this site exists. If they claim to have operated for years but they have been online for 3 days, simply **skip them**. You can research a domain for the amount of traffic it receives at www.alexa.com. If a site is one of the top 100,000 from hundreds of millions in Internet, it is definitely **trustworthy**.

What about little known companies, web sites and supplements? It is quite simple. Let's say that I invest a few thousand dollars in a capsules-making machine and buy huge amount of individual minerals and vitamins at wholesale prices. I mix them as a single product, let's say "Vitamagic", and sell it through my own web site. This is "dietary supplement". This automatically means that FDA will not regulate it for content, purity or quality.

I personally have no intention to have my own company or any affiliations. This is the only way to be **100% loyal to you** and to your best interest. Then and only then can I confidently tell you "only the truth" without hiding or exaggerating absolutely anything to the best of my knowledge.

Testosterone and Low Serotonin- Potentially Deadly Combination

Will you believe that every decent and moral man can easily become a **merciless killer**? Believe it or not this is a fact which has already changed criminal stereotypes and even court sentences. How is it possible? The reason is the potentially deadly combination of severe Serotonin deficiency and high testosterone. Let's explore it in details. Serotonin is an important neurotransmitter and has a crucial inhibitory role on the conversion of Dopamine into Adrenalin. Every one quickly goes into "Fight or Flight" state without it.

Take for example my nearly fatal case. The over ejaculations and restricted food intake had depleted my Serotonin levels while the regular masturbations had boosted the testosterone levels. At the end I almost killed myself. You cannot clearly evaluate the situation and your behaviour when this particular biochemical frame governs your brain, mind and body. That's why there are men who kill people and in the court clearly confess it. However, they also describe this weird mindset and the associate feelings.

People who take Ecstasy are especially vulnerable to becoming dangerous to themselves or to people around them. Severe Serotonin deficiency occurs within 24 hours because of the full release of this substance in the blood and the impossibility of the regulating mechanism to store the excess.

Young men, who mainly take Ecstasy, very often have sex while they are under its influence which seriously boosts their testosterone levels. As a result, on the next day they can easily become very aggressive (fight state).

Even a reproof for a small thing can easily enrage this person and later on force him into murder. In such case, Serotonin is the missing break in the behaviour, while the role of testosterone is to energize the impulses which arise in the person. If they are for sex, the testosterone will urge you to really make it even if it is a rape. If the impulse is to kill another person, it will make you do it. Testosterone itself is neutral and harmless. The problem comes from the nature of the impulses it gives you power and determination to execute.

Several studies and criminal statistics show that when there is severe Serotonin deficiency, the rate of serious crimes such as attacks, rapes and murders is proportionate to the levels of testosterone. In men it is highest between 16 and 30, which is exactly the age of most criminals.

Do you have outbursts of anger or mood swings, which are difficult to control? Then first and foremost increase the level of Serotonin in your body. After that it will be safe to increase your testosterone levels. If you break this sequence, the situation becomes exactly when you drive fast without having reliable breaks. The crash is **guaranteed**. This biochemical combination will either hit you (flight state) or other people (fight state). In both cases, you will **not** be in control of yourself and will surely be sorry later.

Some of the killers instead of execution sometimes get life sentences because of the presence of such biochemical abnormalities. However, is it worth to spend all your life in a prison because of low Serotonin levels when it is quite easy to prevent it? I think **no** and a diet including (whey) protein and if necessary pharmaceutical grade 5-HTP, will keep you away from having such problems.

There is one more thing you can do regarding Serotonin. The level of love and care towards your children when they are still very young determines the level of active Serotonin in their bodies throughout their whole life. That's why hug and kiss them as much as possible. Show them how much they mean to you and they will grow happy, energetic and aggression/depression-free.

Testosterone and Sex

2 years ago, I was passing by a TV set and one of the lawyers from Ally McBeal was obviously in a tough situation after a confession. It impressed me so much that I stopped and watched. "I prefer to pay to a prostitute instead of taking a girl from a bar and have sex with her. I don't have feelings towards them. That's why I consider it fairer to pay for the service of a prostitute." Well, this was very strong scene and it reflects one of the most common problems, which men face regularly. No wonder that prostitution is considered "the most ancient profession".

Personally, I have never considered going to a prostitute. Probably I was lucky to have already sex toys "like-real-flesh" especially molded to the smallest detail from the "mega porn stars of all times". From moral point of view, they are definitely preferable, cheaper and 24 hours a day available for you.

Then comes the question for the importance of daily sexual activity. Here are the fascinating results from just one study. It actually caused a fundamental change in my perceptions about sex, testosterone and health. During the study, the testosterone levels of men who had sex for

11 nights increased. On the contrary, the testosterone levels of the other men who **did not went down.**

So let's say that going to a prostitute is OK for you. Suppose that you spend at least $100 for a girl every day. This will cost you $3,000 only the first month and you will have sex only once per day. Will you enjoy the testosterone (and pleasure) benefits documented at this and other studies? Surely. Is this affordable for the average man? Definitely not! Will most men like the idea to have daily sex with prostitutes? I don't think so, because they will start to question their ability to attract a lady. It seems that the prostitutes are in the best case too expensive way to keep your testosterone levels high on a daily basis. What are the alternatives?

The first thing, which comes to my mind, is to manage alone as many men do. However, the superiority of (regular) sex over masturbation has already been scientifically proven. That's why I strongly recommend the following to every single man. Invest time, energy and money to build a strong, good quality and lasting relationship with a woman, instead of hoping or relying on after-a-bar/one-night shots. This will build your self-image as a gentleman with high moral, health/safety consciousness and sense of responsibility. On other hand, this is better for the overall quality and quantity of sex you will enjoy- an exemplary **win-win situation**.

Is it easy to find and attract a good girlfriend? I wish it were, but in reality sometimes it takes **months** before you meet a lady and there is a big sparkle of biochemistry between you. Then let's say that you have succeeded and you have a girlfriend, fiancée or even wife. Is it easy to convince her to have sex with you every 365 days/year? I don't know about you, but I haven't achieved it yet.

Let's say that you are some Sex God and you have sex with your lady every single day. Is this everything you can do for your ultimate sexual and overall health and anti-aging? Not at all. If this surprises you, then you should know that the real "fountain of youth" for men is **Luteinizing hormone - Testosterone - Sex**.

This specific combination and topic is both crucial and huge. That's why I only started it here and will dedicate a BIG chapter to it in my next advanced book "Your Scientific Diet for Men". It will receive so much attention, because testosterone plays a **key role** in the building and maintaining of a lean and athletic body throughout your whole life.

Master Plan for Men's Ultimate Pleasure and Sex

As you have seen so far, everything narrows down to **knowledge**. If you have it, the result is multiple orgasms, ultimate sexual performance 24/7/365 and minimum risk of common male health problems. That's why my first piece of advice is to <u>keep educating yourself</u>. The more you know, the better quality your whole life will be.

In this book, the focus is on achieving and enjoying ultimate sexual performance, health and pleasure **throughout your whole life**. For the best possible sex, the condition, performance and abilities of **your partner** are of equal importance. That's why I will come up with an equivalent of this book "Scientifically Guaranteed Female Multiple Orgasms and Ultimate Sex®".

There are certain substances such as **Acetylcholine, Serotonin, Dopamine** and **L-Arginine**, which similarly play a very important role in women. There are several other substances, which are specific for them and are the male's equivalent of testosterone, 5-alpha-reductaze, NO and cGMP. I am very happy that there are increasing number of formulas, which supply many of all necessary substances for **ultimate female** sexual performance, health and pleasure.

If you are a middle-aged man and have the impression that your lady's vagina is getting looser, this is quite possible. While men suffer from **penile shrinkage** after 40, women's vaginas **loose**. The result is the sexual crisis couples go through in their middle age. Additional factor is poor or superficial <u>preparation</u> of the vagina for sex. Any forced or aggressive stretching or dry rubbing will speed up the process of loosening and <u>damaging</u> of the delicate tissues, blood vessels and nerves in her vagina. This is definitely **not** in your or her interest.

Another <u>very bad practice</u> is to use **saliva** as a lubricant. First, it contains millions of bacteria, which can cause her **infection**. That's why is imperative to brush your teeth with an **anti-bacterial toothpaste** before having (oral) sex. Second, saliva dries within a few minutes and cannot substitute the natural lubricants, which a carefully warmed and stimulated vagina produces.

Especially when you have a partner, cleaning your **tongue** every morning is <u>essential</u>. You have to see with your own eyes **several brown layers** going out for 2-3 minutes while you clean it with a very gentle pressure of a teaspoon. They contain <u>huge amounts</u> of toxins, bacteria and waste products, which your body has excreted. Now imagine the following common scene.

A man wakes up in the morning with a fully loaded erection. He gently opens the legs of her partner and starts licking her vagina's opening with his **brown tongue** and secreting/spitting on it **biohazardous saliva**. This is enough to make my hair stand on end! If you go in the morning to a prostitute, will you take a shower, brush thoroughly your teeth with an anti-bacterial toothpaste and clean your tongue with a teaspoon? **I doubt it.**

That's why if your lady means something to you, then she **definitely deserves** to get every day the <u>very best</u> of you! Both of you have to maintain perfect hygiene every single day of your life, with **no exceptions**. This is the best foundation of a committed and healthy sexual relationship. I will provide full details on how women can tighten their vaginas, multiply their pleasure and orgasms, and why fisting and anal sex are <u>very bad</u> for them in "Scientifically Guaranteed Female Multiple Orgasms and Ultimate Sex".

"Educational" Sex Video Series versus Porn

I deeply believe that having a fantastic sexual life on a daily basis is of <u>paramount importance</u> and science already backs it up. At the same time, the "educational" sex books and DVDs at the world's market are of **very poor quality**. For example after seeing so many ads of The Better Sex video series, I finally decided to see what is so great about them that "4 million people" have bought them. This was one of my greatest disappointments. In the ads, I see hot young couples almost doing passionate sex in front of my eyes.

In reality, **50%** of the time is dedicated to... sitting and talking general stuff and things like that. When it comes to action, in **50%** of the cases it is performed by **elderly overweighed couples** with gray/white hair and the men are nearly or completely impotent. That's why **80%** of the real action is limited to stripping, kissing, hugging and massaging. I would say that such "educational" videos are good for newbies. However, will teenagers watch foreplay of unattractive elderly couples? I doubt it.

After the successful creation of this book, I already consider to do something in this direction as well. For example, in the near future I intend to write 2 instructional sex books of high quality. However, it is quite difficult for a man to write in full details and cover successfully both **fellatio** and **cunnilingus**. That's why I also consider teaming up with my **hot sister Nadya Ritz**.

The majority of customers who have bought "sex educational" books and video series complain that they:

- **provide no new information**
- most of the time someone is sitting and talking
- unprofessional (very low budgeted and poorly shot)
- **nothing up-close and really instructional**
- unattractive actors
- very short duration or small quantity of information
- boring

Fucking versus Love Making- A Solution to the Modern Crisis of Manliness and Spontaneous Sex

I am 100% sure that even if a couple has the best sexual education in the world it **may not really matter**. What do I mean? I agree that for thousands of years women had had actually **no right** to do something more than look after the children and satisfy the sexual needs of their husbands. Whenever he wanted, she simply had to undress and to spread her legs without any objection.

However, during the last 90 years the situation has changed **completely**. For the short period 1914-1945 (31 years), due to the First and Second World Wars **72 million** people, mostly men, died. This severe and sudden shortage had to be compensated mainly by women. They had to do more and more jobs traditionally held only by men. This has gradually built their confidence, self-esteem and financial independence. Soon women's emancipation and feminism began and sent the old-fashioned stereotypes, especially those, regarding sex, in the history.

Nowadays I can say that women witness their revenge. Men **have to be** "romantic", "gentle", "patient" and especially to **love to** "make love". Sex has become more or less a dirty word. If a man, who has had a long enough relationship with a woman, is in the mood for an old-fashioned fucking right now and right there, he... **cannot** go for it! Why? There is nothing "romantic" in it. He has to go the established route of at least either 15 minutes of kissing, hugging, massaging, etc. foreplay or **suppress** his spontaneous sexual impulse.

More and more men force on themselves such sexual censorship, which is very bad for them. And the result is that there are more than **30 million impotent men** only in the USA! Several years ago, I read the results of a survey, which found out that around <u>50%</u> of the American men preferred **working extra hours** instead of having sex! I could **not** believe my eyes!

However, there is a very sound biochemical reason- testosterone's negative feedback. The less sexually active is a man over a period of time, the <u>lesser he becomes</u> as a result from the gradual decrease in the production of sex related hormones. This is a horrible, but a completely logical and expected consequence from the entire tendency towards sex nowadays.

Is there a light in the tunnel? **Definitely** and we the men should **not** pay for what our grandfathers and grand grandfathers had done. Personally, I am a committed supporter of a <u>win-win and balanced</u> sexual relationships. First, **you give her what she wants** by making love together most of the time. Then, **she gives you what you want**. 1-2 times per month to go straight to the point and make 100% sex even if it is on the kitchen table. Of course, you still <u>must</u> take care of her and her body especially by using **a lot of lubricant** to compensate the lack of foreplay.

My experience with women proves the following thing. After **at least 3 months'** relationship when you clearly state this win-win situation, **99%** of them will agree. Then after 2-3 weeks of "love making" when the testosterone in you surges and it is time for a **quickie, enjoy it**. It is also an opportunity for them to unleash their animalistic female nature, which is equally passionate and adventurous.

A small part of them, who are more feministic, refuse to do anything, which is **not pure** "love making". If I find out such woman and hear her demands for a **win-lose sex game,** I escort her to the front door and close it behind her. Definitely, a modern man should NOT fuck all the time! Our male nature pops up less than **3 times per month**. Then you should have already negotiated a win-win deal with her, which gives you a green light for **just sex at the spot**.

A Major Proof for "Life is unfair!"

Human beings do **not** have a mating season. That's why women expect from us to be able to get an erection 24 hours a day 365 days per year. Is that fair? Not at all. Then we also have to raise the bar accordingly. During the **first 3 months** of a relationship, I do **not** talk or have sex with her. There are so many other things, which are of higher priority for a blissful and long-lasting relationship.

150

In the cases when everything is all right, I voice my requirement for a **regular sex for at least 10 minutes**. The second thing I negotiate about is a **quickie** for 1-2 times per month. What she gets is dedicated, top quality "love making" every time. So far, **100%** of my girlfriends have found this "sex deal" completely "fair" and have complied with it. I can assure you that it is exactly a win-win situation, which helps the relationship to **flourish**.

Women are biologically programmed to search for an **"Alpha Male"**. If they succeed to put a leg on your neck you will **NOT** be such man! That's why it is very important to defend all your natural needs, including the sexual ones, with <u>strong arguments</u>. Such an open communication will help you to win her respect.

It is still more common the man in a couple to be better paid and with a higher social position than the woman. This can lead to uncertainty and even desire in her to **overpower** him. How? By establishing an iron control over his major "switch": **Sex-Testosterone-Health-Wellbeing**.

If a woman keeps your **"switch" off,** then she definitely does her best to arrange for you low quality life and health. I had one such girlfriend and our relationship ended very soon after this.

There are many things, which I can understand and tolerate. It is natural for women to play games and I am used to it. However, I keep in mind the **bare minimum** a man needs from a true win-win relationship and I rarely make compromises!

Unfair but Fact- Hot Women Demand without Caring for Our Natural Limitations

Let's say that you have spent years studying hard at a college for a jump-start at a great career. After that, you have had to prove yourself and **work very hard** to be noticed. And not only that, but you have pushed the iron in a gym to be in top-notch form for years. You have earned enough to buy a house and one day you go out of your stunning car just to meet a **very hot lady**.

Actually, **she bumps into you** and drops her small bag on the ground. As a gentleman, you pick it up and could not help but notice her **long, sexy legs**. She gives you a big, charming smile and apologizes. Her boyfriend has just broken up their 4 months' relationship with a SMS. Now he has a new girlfriend and she is very upset. Touched by her story you ask her whether a dinner at an Italian restaurant will make her feel better. "I guess so" and you go on a date that evening.

There she speaks about your **kindness, tactfulness** and **genuine care**. She shares that "**character**" is what mostly interests her in a man. Gradually you start asking yourself: "Was she going to bump into me if I

- did **not** have a luxury car
- wore an old T-shirt and jeans instead of a suit
- was not in a good shape

When it comes to women in great part of the cases, there is **no** such think as a "coincidence". They select consciously or unconsciously who to bump "incidentally" into and who to pass by. If everything on you and in your possession does not scream "**Alpha Male**", the chances to attract the attention of a hot girl are nearly zero. Fortunately, many men achieve it. However, only they know what they have gone through just to say: "I did it!" Dates with hot girls simply follow without even doing something.

However, hot women take it for granted that you are smart, good looking and rich. If you are not, they will **not** waste their time to tell you how important they consider your... "character". If you have made it to **the top,** than you surely have more than enough qualities and talent. If you are high above **the average men,** in the eyes (unconsciousness) of a hot woman your genes are worth considering. That's why for guys at the top it is always easy to wake up next to a nice lady. Let's see what happens in the bed.

If you are a Top Shot compared to the majority of guys, then by default you **must be also a great lover.** Does any woman know that our male bodies are designed and programmed only to fertilize? To a small extend. Do any of them care that we should last up to 90 seconds? **Definitely Not!** What a hot woman will think if a man lasts about 10 minutes? "He may be a top shot but is a poor lover!" However, he has exceeded his natural limit around **10 TIMES!** Who cares? **Not and (hot) women.** Mother Nature has been extremely unfair towards us regarding sex. Should we feel self-pity because of our severe natural limitations? Not at all.

You have put a tremendous amount of efforts to be "outstanding" enough for the inner radar of hot and free girls. Then, after sex with you if they laugh secretly on their way to the next man it will be a personal tragedy for you. We cannot afford to fail at the **last and most important step** from biological point of view- the passing of our genes. For the already successful guys I have developed a Master Plan for Action in this chapter how to score very high in the bed as well.

Oxytocin- the Reason Women should be on a Sexual Diet

Several years ago, I tried to convince an ex-girlfriend in addition to morning sex to help me with the daily 16-20 strokes 3-5 times/day. I explained her thoroughly about the importance of this for maintaining high levels of testosterone throughout the day. What I got was: "If it is so important and takes little, but regular stroking, you can easily use your hand or ultra realistic vaginas". At that time, I did **not** have strong arguments and it was really very demanding.

Later on, I found out clinical studies about 2 little known hormones produced by the pituitary gland- **vasopressin and oxytocin**. This information deepened my viewpoint and approach to sex.

A release of oxytocin in men occurs **exactly before** an ejaculation and <u>generates the orgasms</u>. However, women's pituitary gland releases it even during a stimulation of the clitoris and the vagina's entrance. And what this research show is that **continuous high levels** of oxytocin can negatively affect intelligence and memory! The other hormone **vasopressin** has exactly the opposite effect.

Oxytocin is thought to induce **pair bonding in people**. Levels of oxytocin are found to be higher in people who claim to be falling in love. It is also thought to mediate other forms of pair bonding such as friendship and family relationships. However, people who directly receive this hormone or have continuously elevated levels of it, tend to develop a <u>very strong addiction</u> towards it!

How this information relates to daily morning sex? After a few weeks on such schedule, the big morning shot of Oxytocin in a woman helps to strengthen her bond with you. In addition, it will raise her initiative for morning sex (it occurs just like the mild addiction to a coffee in the morning). During the first week, even if she is reluctant, she will get used to it, due to the burst of oxytocin and its highly pleasurable effect on the body and mind.

In 3 weeks, if you "forget" about your male duties, she will come to you and ask for sex (shot). That's why at first forget about yourself and **focus entirely on her** needs and ultimate experience! In 2-3 weeks, when the mild addiction is already a fact, you will have **100% guaranteed sex every morning.** I wonder how many men in the world can enjoy such pure blessing? My guess is that this is our compensation from Mother Nature.

I have found out that women's requests for "sex" throughout the day are mainly a need for love, closeness and just being together. In such case, I focus on kissing, hugging and romantic talking. I intentionally **avoid** additional direct stimulation of her **genitals and nipples** throughout the day. In this way, constant high levels of oxytocin cannot be maintained.

Women who are **not** on such "sexual diet" can easily become **airhead nymphomaniacs** (strong addiction + negative effect on their intelligence). In this regard, men may be in a better position, although so many get used to **over-ejaculation**. This surely:

- **ruins** their intelligence
- **shrinks** their testicles
- **slashes** their Testosterone, Acetylcholine, Serotonin, Dopamine and PGE-1 levels
- **severely damages** their overall health

Man can enjoy a lot of sex without worrying about oxytocin by <u>strictly following</u> the recommended ejaculation frequency. This will have strong positive effect on their health. The same has clinically proven **bad** psychological and physiological effect on **women**. As usual, they instinctively know what to do and stay away from too much sex.

Will your Girl Pay $1,000/Night for Your Sex Service

After you learnt the scientific reasons for "women want quality, while man want quantity", let's face the **tough reality**. Would I be able to sleep sound if she does **not** enjoy every single time top quality sex? I don't know for you, but I would not. I want to be one of the very best and in order to achieve it I had to learn from the **best in the world**. That's why a type of guys I still keep an eye on is the professional male escorts. Unbelievably, the good looking and skillful among them get **$700-$1,500 per night!** That's a lot of money for a single hot night, isn't it?

I know exactly what I want from a girlfriend and the only way to get it is to be patient. If I demand on the 2nd day to have sex every morning, my rating can immediately drop to a "pig", "ass hole", "sex maniac", etc. However, if you spend **3 months** with a lady, she will know you quite well. That's why when you finally reach the point to start negotiations for a win-win sex deal, you will be in a **very strong position.** This is extremely important. She trusts you and even more importantly, knows you. So far, I have **successfully closed all sex deals**, which proves that this approach works.

Is your job done if your girlfriend agrees to have sex with you every morning? Oh no, **not at all**. In fact, it has just started. There are **3 billion men,** starting from the guy next door, who are potentially interested in every good looking and sexy girl nearby. That's why logically comes the question. How can you **attract and make loyal** a "good" girl?

Let's make a quick check. You are a "man". So what? You have a penis, testicles and bigger body compared to a woman. Is this a big deal? Not at all, because **3 billion men have the same**. Tell me:

- Why a good girl should pay attention exactly to **you**?
- What **specific** physical advantages do you have compared to 80% of the local men?
- What specific sexual **benefits** can you offer to a girl?
- What specific sexual **experience** can you create for a girl?
- What **little known or advanced** sex techniques can you offer her?
- Why will she want to have sex **again with you to-morrow**?
- What specific benefits and personal advantages do you have that will motivate her to be **100% loyal to you**?

I know that these are tough questions, especially when you ask yourself. Here is the best approach to be able to give **good answers soon**.

Sex Business 101: Sell it to her! Do not tell it to her!

I definitely respect your **sentimental feelings** towards your bulge down there. However, it will **not** attract a hot girl and make her loyal to you. That's why start looking at your penis, testicles, tongue, fingers and body as your

toolbox you use for providing outstanding <u>sex services</u> to a carefully selected lady.

Talking about services, let's say that you want to have a hair cut and accidentally you pass by a **new** hairdressing salon. The shop-window and overall impression is very good. There are no clients and feeling lucky, you enter inside. You open the door, make few steps and freeze. There is hair everywhere, the chairs are old and worn out. The hairdresser gives you a yellow smile and once he comes close to you, you step back disgusted, because he... stinks! Will you leave yourself in the hands of this person? I **doubt it**.

Now scan your memory. Have you ever received a bad service and <u>have gone back</u> for a second one? Most probably **no**. **Why women should react differently?** They neither do it nor will do it! That's why your physical appearance must be the **best advertisement** of "what's in it for me" regarding your outstanding toolbox. Once a girl likes it, she will have a good reason to <u>explore</u> what kind and quality of <u>service</u> you can offer her. If it is equally tempting, you may be <u>hired</u>! If this happens, is it time to relax? **Exactly the opposite!**

You have to <u>prove her</u> that you really deserve the trust she has given you. If you surprise her just like that hairdresser, she will **run away**. And not only this, but she will also **tell all her friends**. Otherwise, she may give you a <u>second chance</u> and come back for more. If you reach this point can you finally lay back and watch TV? Forget about this because while you blissfully stare at the screen, your competition could plan how to attract and steal "<u>your new customer</u>" with a better offer.

If you do **not** believe me, you could ask more than **600** husbands, whose wives were seduced by an **ugly, smelly** and **infected with syphilis** man! Am I joking? Not at all. Let's find out the secret of the greatest female seducer in the history.

The Greatest Secret of Giovanni Casanova

Probably you have heard about **Giovanni Giacomo Casanova** (April 2, 1725 – June 4, 1798) and his sexual adventures. He has described with **pornographic details** each of his affairs in his "Histoire de Ma Vie" (The History of My Life). Uncommonly for his time, he consistently claimed to had been **in love** with all the women he had seduced. Furthermore, he had **never** raped or forced a woman! His greatest secret and major goal had always been to ensure that his partner enjoyed the sex as much as he did.

Well, it may sound quite **simple**, but he had really **done it**. As you know, his fame has continued to live long after he died. Now let's go one step further and find out the **secret behind his** "secret". Can you think of his reason to have sex with more than 1,000 women until his sexual system and health collapsed?

Do you remember the exotic hormone **oxytocin**? Well, Mr. Casanova was nothing more than an oxytocin addict. Everything had started in a religious seminary in Venice where he studied during his teen years. You may be surprised that he was expelled from there for **homosexual acts**! There had been no women and as every teenager, he had had a great sexual rush to satisfy. His adventurous sexual life had forced him all the time either to travel or to hide by going to another town or country.

He got used to **over ejaculations** ever since he was a teenager. During the next decades he had to have sex with an ejaculation at the end just to "get another shot of oxytocin". At the same time this perfectly fits with being "**in love**" with all seduced women. When he had not had a woman nearby, he played with a **male** and even with his **daughter**, with her permission of course.

However, he had paid the price to spend the last years of his life as a **debilitated idiot**. This is due to the effect of oxytocin addiction on the intelligence and of the syphilis. Casanova is a proof from the real life that while women should be on a sex diet, men should be on a **strict ejaculation diet**. Otherwise, both sexes will become obsessed with sex. Have in mind that strong oxytocin addiction can not be cured! The modern medicine can do **nothing** to help people with such problems.

That's why if you find a nymphomaniac, it is better to search for another one. Even if she wants, she will **never be loyal** and satisfied with what only one man can offer her. It is just like to expect from a heroin addict that he will stop taking drugs because of you. It is stronger than they are and once they have started, there is **almost no way back!**

The Daily Testosterone-Boosting Sexual Activity

My usual daily sexual activity consists of two parts. The first one is **30-40 minutes' morning sex**. When I don't have a girlfriend, I use one of the listed below ultra realistic vaginas, which give **99%** of the sensations from real sex. Actually, if I close my eyes, I cannot make a difference because they are made from super hi-tech "like-real-flesh" material!

Then, whenever I am not busy 1-5 times throughout the day, I make 16-20 thrusts in one of them. I **never** make more because my goal is to cause a spike in my body's Luteinizing hormone (LH)-testosterone production. If I continue, my body will start producing a lot of NO/cGMP and 5-alpha-reductaze for DHT conversion. I do not need this. The point is just to trick your body that you are going to have sex so it will immediately take actions to boost the testosterone levels.

There is **another way** to maintain your LH-testosterone levels high. However, it requires taking 2-3 pills every day. Regarding this approach I use a patented brand with thorough clinical studies and excellent proven results. I will discuss this option in "Your Scientific Diet for Men", because maintaining high testosterone levels **through-out your whole life** is of <u>crucial</u> importance to look and feel great. Both ways deliver and can synergistically work together. When you have more free time, for example weekends, you may prefer the sexual boosting. When you are very busy throughout the day, 1-2 pills can pro-duce the same effect.

For the average guy it takes **many years** to find and get married for the lady with capital L in his life. Does this mean that we have to just dream about regular sex until we "make it"? From scientific point of view, such scenario is <u>very bad</u> for our health, confidence and even success in life.

Human beings have spent **95%** of the time in a **Stone Age** environment and lifestyle. Let's see a typical day from that time. After a more or less successful hunting, the male seeks the intimate company of his female. This is a <u>natural and important way</u> to boost his testosterone levels, confidence and motivation to fight with the severe life for both of them.

Back in 21 century we, men, **do not need less** the benefits of daily sex. After a demanding or challenging day, **5-10 minutes' sex** will clear your mind, calm down the stress and help you switch to a very positive mindset for the rest of the day. If you have a girlfriend or a wife, is it a good idea after the morning sex to seek her intimate company? **Definitely no** and you already know why. That's why even if I have a lady I do **not** ask her for sex after the morning. The only exception is 1-2 times/month when I am nuts about a female.

Scientific Breakthrough Every Man should Use

There has been a **scientific breakthrough** for the last few years, which allowed the production of **"ultra realistic" sex toys**. Moreover, they are molded on the "greatest porn actresses of all times". The result is an exact replication of the entire intimate parts of women **to the smallest details**, which are <u>physically perfect</u>. I have very poor knowledge of porn stars. That's why if you are more familiar with this, the **top 10 replicated stars** are:

- Jenna Jameson
- Tera Patrick
- Devinn Lane
- Briana Banks
- Dasha
- Devon
- Lexus
- Sky
- Stormy

From 100's of female porn stars these are referred everywhere to as **the best of the best** so I guess it is true. I have zero interest towards their qualities as actresses.

However, when it comes to exact ultra realistic rep
tions, the models **do matter**.

I have spent a total of **1.5 weeks** browsing through more
than **one thousand sex toys in Internet**. I can confidently say that I have seen the good, the bad and the
ugly. Believe me there are sex dolls, which are **so disgusting** that you can have nightmares especially if you
buy one of them. Psychologically driven erectile dysfunction is guaranteed because even a desperate for sex man
has some minimal requirements.

Here is the place to state that this book, together with
any additional, are appropriate for people on a shoestring
budget. One of my objectives is to **save you money!**
However, there are **3 areas** where even if you are really
on a very tight budget, you have to find a way to get yourself <u>the very best</u>. They are:

-   bed and bed linen
-   underwear
-   ultra realistic sex toys

I will provide several exhaustive lists with **the very best
options** in these areas. Then it is up to you, your taste
and budget. You will probably notice from my lists that
there are **not** anatomical replications made of latex, silicon, jelly or rubber. A modern man who demands the
very best uses **only** exact replications made of any of the
following 6 breakthrough materials:

-   Cyberskin
-   UR3 (ultra realistic version 3)
-   Virtual touch
-   Pleasureskin
-   Passionskin
-   Futurotic

What these materials have in common is that they provide **ultra realistic feeling** on touch and penetration. Of course, there are subtle differences among them and it is already a personal choice what you will like better. What I can assure you is that they all are **fantastic**. The lists below are in random order and provide the exact official names even if there are vulgarities or misspellings in them. You can use them as keyword phrases for example at www.google.com. Let's start with the **top 15 pocket size** ultra realistic masturbators-vaginas.

- Jenna Jameson Pocket Pal
- Passionskin cock stroker
- Cyberskin Pussy Pocket Pal
- Sunrise UR3 Pussy Pocket Pal
- Eve's Pleasureskin Pussy Natural/Cinnamon [colour]
- Tawny Roberts Red UR3 Pocket Pal
- Tera's Futurotic Stroker Bonanza
- Tera Patrick's Futurotic Stroker
- Pleasureskin Cheap Sex
- Jessica Drake's Futurotic Pocket Pal
- Cyberskin Cyber Pussy
- Jana's Futurotic Pussy
- Devon's Private Pleasures
- Aria's Body Stroker Futurotic Masturbator
- Cindy Crawford Cyberskin Pussy

The price range online is **$20-$28**. There is a great selection and they are very affordable even for a shoestring budget. You can place a pocket pal on your penis and move it with your hand(s) up and down. Another option is to wrap it with a heavy towel for example for a **hands free** action. In both cases the sensation is exactly as if you have sex. Talking about masturbators, you should carefully consider 2 things. The first one is a high quality lubricant. Just like with a real vagina, you can **not** get directly inside because the rubbing will be quite unpleasant.

Second, <u>match the size</u> of your penis with the masturbator. If the circumference of your penis is 6 inches, this means you need a pocket pal with minimum **2 inches in diameter**. If a replication is only 1 inch in diameter, you will tear it. They are **not stretchy** beyond the stated diameter. Personally, I will never buy a masturbator without knowing its **length and diameter**. If it is not written clearly on the web site, look for another one or **ask** their customer service. It is useless to pay for something, which does **not** fit you good enough to provide the sensations of a real sex.

The effect on your body from using any of the top quality masturbators mentioned above is **much greater** than simply using your hand and fingers. In fact, the old-fashioned masturbation usually leads to <u>curvature</u> because the majority of guys use mostly one hand. Moreover, it is **not** easy or comfortable to stroke an upright erection. That's why unnoticeably the palm **curves the penis** to the left or right and downward or upward. It is very easy to know a man's preferred hand and technique for masturbation exactly from the curvature of his penis.

All ultra realistic toys made from the top 6 materials are soft and gentle on touch. However, upon pressure you will feel a **hard layer** below the surface just like the real thing. That's why it is **impossible** to curve your penis and in this way to damage it using any ultra realistic replication. It is a must for <u>every</u> sexually healthy and mature man to have at least one pocket pal because they are fantastic and very affordable.

Once a male reaches sexual maturity around 14, it is better and healthier to get used to **realistic** and **visu-**

ally pleasing female replication(s) instead of his hand. Regarding a purchase for a teenager, I think that Jenna Jameson Pocket Pal is **not** a good option because it looks a little bit strange from the outside. The others are **perfect** for this purpose.

What every man **must always use** in addition to a sex toy is lubricant. A long time ago on the market popped up **water based lubes**. However, they <u>dry within minutes</u>. Once you begin to feel great pleasure and increase the number of strokes or penetrations, the last thing you will think of is to lubricate your love tool. However, dry rubbing is **the best way to damage** the very delicate skin of your penis and break many blood vessels.

If this happens, you have to supply liquid **Vitamin E** and rich in **Gamma-linolenic acid** oil to boost locally the levels of Prostaglandin E-1. Otherwise, the released collagen will cause <u>scar tissues</u> at the places of the damages. In the long term, the surface of your penis can become **very** bumpy, deformed and ugly. To avoid such possibility here is the **keyword phrase** for the only type of lubricant a modern man should use:

silicone lubricant -antifreeze -car -metal -water -spray

With any of the brands on the market, all you have to do is put **very little** on your penis or on the walls of a (ultra realistic) vagina and forget about lubricating. They **never dry** and you can have sex even 2 hours without any possibility for a damaging dry rubbing. In addition, they match with and perfectly protect all hi-tech and top quality sex toys I have listed.

The mineral **silicon** itself is a part of many multi mineral formulas so it is **edible**. On the contrary, half of the ingredients of all water soluble lubes are **preservatives**, which are not good for the health. Even with their presence, they can do almost **nothing** to stop the evaporation within minutes. Silicon lubricants are next generation and are far superior than any water-based.

Now I can finally list the 3 things, which I **strongly recommend** that every father should provide his 14+ years old son (below his pillow):

- this book
- one of the pocket pals
- 2 big bottles of silicon lubricant

When a young man is <u>very satisfied sexually</u>, he will **hardly** go to an easy female classmate, student or friend. Otherwise, pushed from the huge testosterone peaks and sexual rush, he will readily fuck **the first one he can** as early as 13-15 years of age. Before you argue with me, remember your teen years.

If you have spent some time on teen forums, you will also know what is going on with modern teenagers. It is enough to read posts like: "I am 12 years old guy and I have had sex with 2 girls so far. **Should I feel guilty?**" For me it will be easier to write the comparative analysis of:
- Hydroxyandrost-4-ene-6,17-dioxo-3-THP ether
- delta-4-10,13-dimethyl-cyclopenta[a]phenantrene-3,6,17-trione

for testosterone boosting in "Your Scientific Diet for Men" than to answer such posts. Nowadays, teens need <u>a lot of</u> support, information, understanding and faith that they will take the right decisions.

I suppose that some men and fathers will never consider a realistic replication of a female vagina. I certainly understand and respect your position. In this case, **very friendly** for conservative men and still heightening your pleasure are the following 5 options:

- Colt Gear Hand Job Stroker
- Jac off silicon glove
- Hand Job Stroker
- Ultimate Jack Off Sleeve
- Variations Hummer Masturbator

Now let's move forward towards the best "**girlfriend in need**" for every 16+ man- the ultra realistic intimate parts of a physically perfect female. It is pleasure for me to present you the following **top 10**. There are many others, but it is unbelievable how ugly most of them are. If you see and try any of the perfect molds below, you will **never** masturbate the old-fashioned way or be sorry for not having a girl for some time! I guarantee you. Many guys write that it is even "**better than my girlfriend**"!

As you know, I follow a very strict policy towards recommendations. The only reason to show some enthusiasm here is that **sometimes** the pleasure from sex with one of the top 10 is really better than the real thing. They are that unbelievably good! You have to see for yourself how almost **surrealistically perfect** they look (and feel). However, I always aim at something **more than sex**. That's why a replication will never replace a real woman.

Two of the listed below are for **doggy style** sex (access from behind) while the rest are for **missionary position style** (access from their front).

- Devinn Lane's Vibrating Double Pleasure
- Jenna's Vagina and Ass
- Tera Patrick pussy and ass (doggy style)
- Jenna's Vibrating UR3 ass and pussy (doggy style)

- Briana Banks Pussy and Ass
- Lexus Ultra Realistic Vibrating Vagina and Anus
- Devon UR3 Vibrating Pussy and Anus
- Sky UR3 Vibrating Vagina and Anus
- Stormy Vagina And Anus
- Dasha's Squirting - Vibrating UR3 Vagina and Anus

Note: Are you used to water-based lubricants and have a serious reason not to upgrade to the non-drying silicon ones? In this case **Dasha's** tight vagina and anus may be the best option. You can fill the squirting ball with lube. Then from time to time squeeze it and your penis will be lubed up again without having to stop thrusting. If the issue is a tight budget then this replication is also cheaper than most of the others. Regarding its quality I have read only positive comments about it.

It is true that the 2 doggy style exact replications are nearly **twice as expensive** as the missionary ones. However, they are the most visually mesmerizing, surrealistically perfect and in the long-term the pleasure pays off. After all, they are molded on the **only two "megastars"**, while the other eight are only "**superstars**".

Back to your son, a pocket pal will most probably do the trick for **1-2 years**. That's why at his 16<u>th</u> birthday it is time for **more**. The only substitute of real female's private treasures is an ultra realistic exact replication. If you do **not** provide such to him, he will **go and find a real one**. Otherwise, he will be busy with an **outstanding replication**, which will keep him **very** sexually satisfied. That's why for sure he will take his time to find a good young lady.

The whole plan up to here is **the only one**, which really gives gradually to your son <u>what he needs when he needs it</u>. In addition, he will **not** face an overwhelming need to start having sex with women before becoming an adult at 18. The strongest and last indicator that he already considers sex is to date girls. Then it is already **urgent** to provide him this option. It is especially important for him to think and takes decisions with his <u>upper head</u> and **not** with his lower head. Also men are more confident, patient and **date better** when they have a **solid** (sexual) back up.

Let's continue with the next list. I am well aware that 99.9% of all men **love oral sex**. That's why for the lonely periods here are 5 options:

- Tera Patrick Succulent Cherry Mouth
- Cyberskin Cyber Sucker
- Hustler Lip Service Sleeve
- Perfect Blowjob Mouth
- Cyberskin Twin Teaser

After a small search you can find replication of Jena Jameson's mouth. However, I personally cannot put it on my list because it does **not** deliver outstanding experience. In fact, it can be even unpleasant as if you rub a rubber, which has nothing to do with an oral sex. The numerous others do **not** deserve even to take a glimpse at them.

Regarding other types of sex toys that I do **not** feel comfortable to list is the brand "**Fleshlight**". They are definitely popular, although to get a vagina in a soft drink can is quite eccentric. Moreover, they are proud that their products are **very** or **extremely tight**. There is even comparison of the hole with 10 pens coin. So far, the discussion was about "like-real" sex. If you are interested to insert your penis in a keyhole then look around and may find one. After all, what pleasure will you get if you cannot even get inside?

So far I have focused only on the most cherished female anatomical parts for sex. For men who may want a whole "like-real" lady I have only 2 suggestions. They are:

- Tera Patrick's Ultimate Erotic Love Doll
- Jenna's Extreme Dream Doll

Personally, I do **not** have them and I can say nothing about the **experience** they deliver. My selection is based entirely on visual appearance and comparison with all other sex dolls, which are **unbelievably disgusting** and a complete turn off. Just take a look online and you will see what I mean.

These two are quite decent although they are **very expensive**. For about **$340**, Tera Patrick's doll is only nice. Something, which I do not like especially about it, is her **huge breast**. It dominates the whole doll. If you like to have in your hands more than you can handle, she may be good for you. Jenna's doll is around **$100 cheaper** and I was lucky to find a picture after a long search. She looks just like a **Barbie doll**. Great blonde hair, a cute face and still full chest, but **not** too much. I have **not** seen Jenna on DVD, but her doll has great proportions and is "sexy", which is important for an enjoyable sex.

When it is time to talk with a new girlfriend about sex, suddenly in my bedroom appear the following 3 masturbators. They are shaped as a male body with a very cute penis and testicles:

- Soft Touch Male Masturbator
- Nick Manning's Body Slam
- Soft Touch Butt Banger

Girls immediately notice them and soon start caressing their genitals. Is there a better icebreaker than this?

Furthermore, if you want to catch her off-guard and **hear from her** what she thinks about <u>your penis</u> without even seeing it, here is a trick. There are 2 products, which allow to make a **perfect replication** of your love tool. You can even use it after that during sex.

Simply follow several simple instructions and place the result, which looks exactly like a sex toy, in your bedroom. When she looks at it, ask her how it is compared to her ex-boyfriends' love tools. The rest is insider information which otherwise you will never hear from a lady from respect to your ego. Of course, if there is a possibility to get hurt do **not** do it. Here are the available options:

- Make your own dildo kit
- Clone a willy dildo kit

I already listed all sex toys, which can multiply **your** pleasure and sexual activity. The advanced part of the Master Plan that deals with **her** ultimate pleasure will be at "Scientifically Guaranteed Female Multiple Orgasms and Ultimate Sex". You have an important role in it! That's why I will write there a whole chapter **entirely for you**. More specifically, I will list several categories of sex toys, which I call "<u>beta assistants</u>". This is the only way to assist her to experience the **ultimate** in sex. In addition, I will discuss <u>top 12 sex positions</u> and especially the **Master Position**, which I use to give my girl "**the ride of her life**" at the end of each intercourse.

Your Role regarding Female Orgasms

Men can enjoy multiple orgasms due to the **VIP Muscle** and the **Parasympathetic nervous system**. Women on the contrary can achieve the same through intensive, prolonged and simultaneous stimulation of their **Clitoris -**

G spot - Cervix and the **Sympathetic nervous system**. Of course, they also have to maintain their <u>biochemistry in top condition</u>. When you know how, it is very easy to **double** your girl's pleasure without efforts.

Probably you are interested to know my **macro concept** regarding female orgasms. The authors of such books are separated in two extreme categories. Either they demand the lady to take full responsibility of her orgasms or they tie this duty like a big stone on the man's neck. Numerous customer reviews state that neither these approaches work well nor they lead to outstanding sexual experience and multiple orgasms.

Following my unique **scientific-business** approach towards sex, I see your role as the <u>Couple's Orgasms Manager</u>. In contrast with the other authors I clearly tell you everything scientifically proven to be important for outstanding sexual abilities, performance and endurance. That's why you can perfectly satisfy your lady by yourself. However, I know from personal experience that no one is in a mood for long lasting multi-orgasmic sex 365 days per year. That's why I provide in the advanced part **additional exhaustive lists** with "beta assistants".

Just like a Manager, you can **delegate** them the "hard work" and see your lady melting from pleasure. Have you seen a Manager to do the entire job in a department? For sure not but it is his primary function to **make sure that the job is done!** Regarding sex, this means that your lady has enjoyed multiple orgasms. It is **not important** whether the majority of them are due to you or your "beta assistants".

In this way, whenever you feel like a "Sex Machine", leave her breathless **yourself**. When you are a little bit lazy leave the "hard work" to your "beta assistants" and only finish her with "the ride of her life" at the end. Regarding it, I insist to be **10 minutes!** If you want more it is fine. If you are healthy, you should be able and willing to have sex for at least 10 minutes every morning. Why is this so important?

First, people remember **the end** of each event. Moreover, you have to maintain your sexual superiority over the beta assistants. These 10 minutes at the end provide sexual stimulation, which is **very** intensive and continuous and generates extreme pleasure and multiple orgasms for her. I will describe **point by point** in the other book how to achieve it.

I think that other authors fail to deliver because they do **not** place themselves in **your shoes**. I regularly do it and that's why there is significant flexibility in my approach. For example, most of my girlfriends wake me up for sex when they are in **ovulation**. On the contrary, when they go through the Post Menstrual Syndrome (PMS) I do **not** wake them up. If she (my alpha female) wants sex in the morning, my default answer is "Certainly, my pleasure". Otherwise, I go to my **ultra realistic beta females**. The last thing I want is to cause my lady pain, which is very possible during the hormonal misbalances after menstruation.

Each rule, which deals with something different from health safety, has exceptions. That's why **actively monitor** your girl and **act accordingly**. Another example is their attitude throughout the month. If she shouts at me during the post menstrual period, I will hug her, kiss her and assure her that I love her and everything is fine. If my hormones are messed up, I will also find it difficult to control my behaviour and emotions. However, if during ovulation she only raises her voice, I will escort her to the front door without blinking. Then she has **perfect**

control over herself and I refuse to tolerate any aggressiveness!

The Good and the Bad Side of "Beta Assistants"

Probably you wonder what these "beta assistants" are. Do I refer to a small army of vibrating, pulsating, rotating, heating and blinking sex toys? **Definitely not** and you will **never** read from me even a suggestion to use such kind of devices. Criterion #1 for me is "naturalness". That's why I did **not** put "Briana's UR3 pocket pussy" on my list. I disqualified it entirely because it is **blue**. As a woman, she is very sexy, the UR3 material is fantastic but you will **not** find in the nature a blue vagina.

The only way for your body to respond in the **most beneficial for you** way is to see and use equivalents as close to the natural as possible. For my regret, most of the **top 15** suggestions for ultra realistic "vagina and ass" have artificial options. **Please, resist using them!** Probably some vibrations, pulsations, etc. effects can give you more pleasure. However, the vagina of **no woman** in the world can vibrate, rotate, blink, etc.

I am glad from the achieved progress in ultra realistic replications. However, they are just like food additives. They should **not** replace the main course.

How do I energize this principle? Once I have a serious reason to break up with a girl, I can use all my beta females for **2 months**. If for that time I haven't found a new girlfriend, I place one of the "vagina and ass" in the wardrobe. After another 2 months if the situation is still the same, I place my second one there as well. Then I can use only few pocket pals but with time, I also place them away. All this **forces me** to keep searching for a great match interested in a serious long-term relationship.

In the following years, I am sure that there will be even better materials, which provide sensations that are even more realistic and probably superior than real sex. However, I consider all of them "beta" or **deputy** in my sexual hierarchy. I will **always remain loyal** to having sex with a real, breathing lady. Only such one can have "alpha status". If the manager of a department leaves, the deputy takes over. However, this is always **temporary** until a new leader is hired.

Why should be different with sex partners? If you split up with your girlfriend or wife (for some time), you have the beta assistants. They will take care for your sexual needs. Once you are again with a lady, they automatically move to a **secondary position**. A replication can keep you sexually satisfied day after day.

However, even the toughest men out there needs to be **loved** deep inside him. An artificial sex toy can **never** kiss you, hug you or tell you "I will remember this night for the rest of my life." I do believe that every man needs these things. That's why the progress should **never** distract us from being interested and loyal to the real things. If you get used to some artificial effects then the sex with a real woman will **never give you great satisfaction**. At the end, you will become a **slave** of some piece of hi-tech material.

Another danger is that women use more and more vibrators. This is the **fastest way to damage seriously** the nerves and tiny blood vessels in their genitals! Just think about the nature of these vibrations for a while. If you put your chick next to a vibrator, the feeling is quite unpleasant. Why? You will feel **powerful mini shockwaves**. On a larger scale give yourself several very quick punches in the chick and tell me whether you enjoyed the experience. For millions of years the female vagina has reached a **perfection to withstand thrusts**.

However, the huge number of shockwaves from modern vibrators reaches "hyper-sonic" levels. Now imagine 100s of powerful shockwaves hitting every minute the ultra delicate and <u>unprotected</u> nerves and tiny blood vessels in the vagina. Unfortunately, once they are damaged it is **difficult to heal** them. That's why **make sure** that you and your girl stick only to <u>natural</u> beta assistants, speeds and ways to have sex. The rest in one way or another **will damage** your genitals, bodies and pleasure!

Your Sexual Territory- Your Rules and Superiority

My Master Plan also makes it **legitimate for her** to experience other penises (some of the beta assistants). However, let's say that your penis is **5.5 inch in length**. Imagine that you buy "John Holmes Ultra Realistic cock", which is **12 inches** and you give it to her. She looks at it and then looks at your penis, which is **not even half** of it. What would she think about your love tool? The chances are that it will **not** be something positive.

Women do compare and the odds in their game **always** have to be <u>in your favour</u>! That's why here is a crucial <u>Iron Rule</u>: "Never allow an imitation of a penis to be longer or thicker with **0.5 inches** than your own penis! Otherwise, you will simply <u>humiliate yourself</u> in front of her! Let's say that it is **not** John Holmes's but a common 8 inches dildo. If she gets used to it and all you can naturally offer her is 5.5 inches, which is above average, you may **get a problem**. Today will be the toy you gave her. Tomorrow can be the penis of the guy next door, which is longer and/or thicker than yours.

For this reason comes <u>Iron Rule N2</u>: "Your own love tool must give her the **greatest pleasure** compared to any other sex toy (beta assistant)." **No exceptions!** If she needs a longer penis, then definitely use the scientific knowledge from this book to restart the enlargement from your teens. Of course, keep the limit of **7 inches** in your mind. Anything more is <u>against your best interest and health</u>!

Genetics versus Religion and Moral- My Solution

As males, we are genetically programmed, which has also been scientifically proven, to be <u>polygamous</u>. This means that we have to have and fertilize **more than one female**. Despite this, I demand from myself to be 100% loyal to my alpha female (girlfriend). As you already know, when 3 months have passed and a girl is still with me it is time for "let's talk about sex, baby".

First we negotiate the frequency. Then I show her my 2 ultra realistic exact replications, which I personally like the most from the top 15 above. The reactions are mixture of surprise, amazement at their "incredibly realistic" look and feel on touch and a little bit jealousy. "Do you often fuck them?" This is an excellent opportunity to explain her thoroughly the benefits for my testosterone production of regular sex shots throughout the day. In addition, I tell her about **oxytocin** and why she should **avoid** asking me for sex more than once a day.

From the feedback I receive, I always score many points for knowing such "advanced" information and being so "genuinely concerned" about her health and well-being. This is the second chance for me to state that I target a "win-win situation" in everything and they believe me. Exactly 1 week after we start having sex it is time for a **preplanned provocation**.

While she enjoys great pleasure I stop, take out a replication and with a **big smile on my face** start fucking it while looking my girl in the eye. The reaction is always from a controlled to a quite sharp. This is exactly what I want from her. Once I get it I immediately raise my voice. Then with an angry look and looking her right in the eye tell her:

- I expect to see **your appreciation** that I am trying to diversify my sex life with some stupid female imitation in front of you instead of **fucking now another girl behind your back!**
- (after a few speechless seconds with starry eyes) Yes...yes, of course! I do appreciate that you are so honest and loyal to our relationship. Thank you very much for this. As you told me before, the feeling with them is 99% like a real sex so I do hope that you enjoy it. Please continue. I will wait.
- Enough. I have something much better (and jump again on her)!

So far, I have never received a second objection for having sex with my 2 beta "girls". Out of respect towards my **alpha female,** I avoid taking them out while I am with her. The only exception is when the testosterone levels in me change a gear.

One of my ex-girlfriends after this standard for me "angry scene" jumped on my neck, kissed me and said: "Some of my ex-boyfriends told me looking me in the eye that I am the best woman they had ever dated. Few weeks or months after that I caught them with other women. You can hardly imagine how **betrayed and depressed** I felt for weeks after each of these incidents. Now you are cheating me in front of me but I am actually happy and thankful. I can see that it is just sex with this "girl" and I can easily "share" you sexually with "her". Now I trust you more than ever. After all, the most important is that your heart and mind are interested and loyal only to me. I am very happy and proud to be your **'alpha'** female."

Definitely, it takes a great deal of **honesty, respect** and **win-win thinking.** The aim is <u>both</u> of you to get what you want without breaking your relationship or compromising with your needs and desires. What I initially wanted to achieve is to **legitimize** my male genetic programming. I realized long time ago that no matter what I try, **I will never change it.**

I am deeply religious, very moral and at the same time, I need to have sex on a weekly basis with 2-3 girls. Could you advise me who I may go to and complain about this **absurd situation**? God is high, the Pope is far and as usual, I had to find a win-win solution myself. That's why I am so happy that I neither have to lust secretly other girls nor to cheat behind her back. So far, each of my girlfriends has had nothing against this situation. In fact, they are happy that I am **very sexually satisfied** and actually have <u>zero reasons</u> even to think for another girl.

Imagine the following situation. Every single morning for the last 1 year, you have had a **bow with oatmeal for breakfast**. One day you go to a friend's house and see a packet of oatmeal. From first sight, it catches your eye and you start dreaming how much you will enjoy even if you could taste only 1 spoon from it. You wait for the host to go out for a while and jump on the oatmeal. It is so

marvelous that you eat it until the last piece. Is there any chance such scenario to happen in reality? I doubt it.

If you have oatmeal for breakfast every day and see somewhere a packet, I doubt that you will pay any attention to it. Why? You have reached **the point of saturation**. You enjoy your morning oatmeal but you do **not** look around for more. The same is with sex and women. If you are **very satisfied** from your sexual life with a girl you love and admire, the **last thing** you will consider is to seduce other women or cheat on her.

Probably you will **not** be surprised that women are genetically programmed to be **monogamous**. That's why it is difficult for them to understand common men's statements such as "It was only sex". However, if you open a newspaper or go on a site with personal classified ads, you can often read: "married woman seeking a discreet affair. 555-555-555" If it is difficult for them to stay loyal, it is at least **10 times** more difficult for us. However, this is **NOT an excuse** to fuck around while having a relationship!

My Health Safety Policy Regarding Oral Sex

You spend some time with a new girlfriend and gradually end up having sex. I do hope that you **always put a condom** on your penis. What interests me is do you have oral sex with her? Do you lick her clitoris and vagina's opening? If your answer is positive, I can only pray that you are not already infected with HIV/AIDS! In this scenario, the condom has absolutely no way to safeguard you because the **vagina's fluids** of an infected woman are **rich in HIV viruses!** The same is true for the pre-ejaculate fluid of men.

If you are going to tell me something like: "Yes, yes, don't worry. I'll be careful" please **don't!** Here is step-by-step **exactly** what I ask and do with a girl to guarantee myself 100% health safety before I even think for oral sex.

Only after a new girlfriend has lived **3 months** in my house I will consider having any kind of sex with her. Before that **at the end of the 2nd week** together, I ask her few important questions. The first one is:

-   Could you tell me the **exact date** when you had sex for the last time?

If she tells me a specific date, I ask her the **exact time** of the day. I want to be sure that she remembers clearly. Otherwise, if she cannot give me a confident answer I **play it safe** and calculate 6 months from the beginning of our mutual living.

Why do I do this? The **HIV virus** causes a specific reaction from the human immune system. This process can take up to 6 months. Then a reliable HIV blood test can detect it with 100% accuracy. This means that if a girl has **not** had sex for the last 6 months and a blood test shows **HIV negative** for sure she is **not infected**.

The next step is to **learn the degree of trust** you can vote her. For this purpose check her answers against two techniques, which serve as a **verbal detector of truth**. First, you have to find out the time it takes her to give a yes/no answer. Here is a similar dialog:

-   Honey, do you have a headache?
-   **(after 1 second)** No, I feel fine.
-   I want to ask you a very important question and expect a completely honest answer. Are you ready to hear it?

- **(after 1 second)** Yes.
- (looking her at the eyes) Have you ever cheated on your boyfriend?

Now <u>keep your eyes and ears widely open</u>. The **first thing** you have to detect is any **difference in the time for answer** with the default (1 second in my example). If she tells me "no" after **5 seconds** for sure, she <u>has lied on me</u>. This delay of 5 times is the time for thoughts like: "Should I tell him? What will he think of me?", etc. This first technique is **very reliable** to expose lies.

If you receive a negative answer use again this technique by asking for confirmation:

- Are you sure?

Again, pay special attention to any difference **greater than 2 seconds** in the time for response.

The second technique is used by **CIA agents** with estimated 80% accuracy. While telling you "no", if you see <u>horizontal wrinkle(s) appearing across her forehead</u> it is with 80% certainty that **she has lied on you!** If you have watched the TV statement of Bill Clinton regarding Monica, you could have clearly seen deep wrinkles appearing on his forehead exactly at the time he said he had had no sexual contact with her.

Consciously, a person can lie very convincingly but such unconscious (**rationally uncontrolled**) signs show to a knowledgeable person what actually **the truth** is. In general, if I see that on the forehead of a person there are deep horizontal wrinkles even without making any face expressions, I never trust them.

Dermatologists have found out that it takes around 15,000 repetitive facial movements to appear a permanent wrinkle. Imagine how many lies a person who has 3 very obvious and deep wrinkles on his forehead have said! I can confidently say that used together, this 2 techniques give **99% accuracy and reliability**.

I had 2 such cases when the girls delayed their response with 3-4 seconds and wrinkled their foreheads. My first reaction was immediately to **escort them to the front door**. One of them wanted to "explain". However, all I wanted to hear is how the front door closes behind her. If you cannot trust <u>100%</u> a girl, none of the condoms and blood tests in the world will guarantee you a long, healthy and happy life.

If her answer comes **without** a delay against the control time **and** horizontal wrinkles on her forehead, I continue.

-    Can I have 100% trust in you?

Once again, a significant delay or wrinkles will show you that she may go to sleep with another guy without telling you. If any of the 2 techniques even hints for a lie, <u>play it safe</u> and immediately **break the relationship**! You can always find another girl. However, if you start having sex and she gets infected while cheating behind your back you **cannot get another life!**

<u>*Never make compromises with your health safety*</u>! Even at the slightest hint that she is **not 100% reliable and trustworthy**, I will be an IDIOT to continue building a relationship with her.

Remember about the 16 years old **Paul** whose girlfriend has "slept around" during their relationship. I am sure that his rational evaluation of her and/or intuition has warned him that she is **NOT trustworthy.** Plus, his father has **not** paid some stupid 20 bucks to provide him a sexual back up in order to have greater resistance towards such obviously "easy girl". Paul has **paid with his life** for over trusting her while his not caring enough father will definitely lead a very unhappy life after attending his **funeral**!

If a lady passes this verbal detector of lies, I explain her about the HIV virus and the 6 months period. Then I offer her a deal. Here is an example:

-   You told me that the last time you had sex was 5 months ago. This means that in 1 month will finish the necessary period for reliable HIV detection. Then I would like **both of us to make a blood test**. I will pay everything. All I want you to do is come with me. In this way both of us will be sure that everything is fine and we can have **safe oral sex**.

Women who are traditionally health conscious eagerly accept my offer and I **score many additional points**. In fact, HIV is **only one** of several health hazards. That's why I request in the hospital the blood to be tested for **Hepatitis as well**. However, there is **no need** to check for syphilis. Its incubation period is **10-90 days** and after that **pink-doted non-itchy rash** appears all over the body. Typical for it is that it pops up also on the palms and feet. If you spend 3 months with a person, you will surely notice such thing.

If the results from the blood test are all **negative,** we can have oral sex. Can you stop being careful? No! Before I have sex for the first time with a new girl, I give her **massage** from head to toe. During it, I make a very close inspection of her body and look for anything suspicious, especially at her genitals. After all, there are more than 5 unpleasant sexually transmitted diseases.

If both this "exam" and the results from the blood test show nothing, then I do **not** think any more about health hazards. If she passes the verbal detectors and I <u>over deliver</u> in the bed, my girl becomes <u>loyal</u>. Then I have **no reasons** to worry about cheating.

Do you see now what really means to "**Think safety first**"? Even if I get married, I will want <u>every year</u> both of us to use at home the only FDA approved anonymous HIV test. It is very simple and the samples go in a laboratory, which makes the results reliable. It costs less than an antivirus program. In contrast with computers, you **cannot buy another life**. If I have children, once they are 13 years old, I will start them on the test as well for my peace of mind. In this way, I will show everyone at home that HIV is something <u>very serious</u> and no one should even think to do **anything**, which can bring him this <u>fatal infection</u>.

Protect and Your Financial Health

What does the latest **Census Bureau report** show about married couples in the USA? "About **50%** of first marriages **for men** under age 45 may end in divorce, and between 44-52% of women's first marriages may end in divorce for these age groups." In Europe, the average is **57%** and reaches **68%** at Russia! As you can see, in half of the cases after some time and despite the great love and mutual admiration at the beginning, **something may go very wrong**.

They get divorced and... the **court usually skins the man alive**. Is this necessary to happen? Should you allow losing **half** of all you have worked so hard to get? Take for example Tom Cruise. Why do you think he got divorced with Nicole Kidman **1 week** before they celebrated their 10th anniversary? He has felt that the time of this relationship has finished or will finish in the near future. In such case according to their preliminary contract, he has to give her **half** of all he has. As a smart men, he arranged the divorce 1 week before the anniversary and they split, which didn't affect his financial status. I wish people paid attention exactly to such **excellent examples** coming from the celebrities instead of spying their private lives.

Moreover, when you break with a lady you need **every bit** of advantage and confidence boost. Why? Because you have to go out and attract **not just** another great lady but a **better one!** If suddenly **half** of what you have disappear, it will hit your confidence when you least need it. I think it is obvious why I am definitely **against** such scenario. That's why set your mind **right from now** on the following topic. Once you find your almost divine Aphrodite, she should sign the dotted line on a carefully though out and discussed contract **BEFORE** you get married. Your financial stability and power in the future will **depend on this with 50% certainty**!

Let her **prove** in this way that she is interested in **you!** And **not** in everything you can offer her **plus** half of your possessions on final farewell. If she gets attracted to another guy, break the marriage and **skin you alive financially,** who will be the love fool. **YOU!** I am sure that you are smart and realist enough to see that relationships often develop in a bad direction. That's why you **must protect** your best interests in advance.

If the situation turns in a court case, the odds automatically become **against you**. Otherwise, with a preliminary contract everything ends up quickly, quietly and <u>win-win</u>. She can go to another guy and you are **still financially powerful** enough to get another great girl.

The smart men in the world <u>think in advance</u> and **never allow** being surprised from easily predictable events. As an **Alpha Male,** let her keep in mind where the front door is and that she can always pack her things and leave your home. Having a preliminary contract is a guarantee that divorce will **not** spell out <u>financial and psychological catastrophe for you</u>!

Life nowadays is stressful enough. That's why make sure to **eliminate any possibilities** to get additional truck-loads of stress from easily preventable events, which do happen. Women are "gentle" creatures but <u>beware</u> if you are soft and gentle with them in such **key aspects**. They will either **kick your ass or step on your neck** if you can offer them a higher standard.

Sex Business 201- Differentiate and Advance Your Sexual Services to "Outsell the Competitors"

Back to the sexual topic, let's say that you have stood out enough from the other guys to make it to the bed. Now could you go on an **instinctive autopilot** and fuck her like an animal? You can but **99.9%** of the other guys can **offer her the same**. If you want to keep her <u>loyal to you</u>, she has to get enough **benefits** from you, which she cannot get from other men.

Take for example this book. Have you ever read anything from the information up to here in another sex-related book or magazine? Surely not, because it is **100% exclusive**. I would **never** win your respect and recommendations if it was "**the same old stuff**" with a new cover. I do my best my girl also to get <u>above 90% exclusive sexual</u> experience. I can assure you that this is a **great loyalty booster**. So far, a serious difference has always occurred in our characters, plans for the future, understanding for life, etc. and we have had to break up.

However, my girlfriends have never done this step first. Even after I tell her that it is obvious that we are **not a perfect match,** they still want to "pass by" (and have sex, of course 100% safe) until one of us finds a new partner. Then after some time they call me back and tell me something like: "My new boyfriend is a great person and man. However, the 15 minutes good fucking he offers me can **not** compare with the professional-grade, highly intensive up to 1.5 hours multi-orgasmic experience with you." Am I born with this knowledge or experience? Definitely not! **Every single man** can achieve all different qualities and abilities I talk about.

You already have the full knowledge how to achieve and maintain your top sexual condition. You also have the full lists with all sex toys, which can increase **your** satisfaction in addition to the VIP Muscle. The rest already deals with her pleasure and how to make sure that she also enjoys every single time ultimate sex. That's why I will explore in full details each of the necessary steps during an **outstanding and memorable intercourse** at "Scientifically Guaranteed Female Multiple Orgasms and Ultimate Sex".

What's next? Crucial Requirements to Reach the Top in Life

It definitely takes **commitment** and **self-discipline** to provide the very best for yourself and your girl **on a daily**

basis. Many guys do **not** make it. That's why they logically witness and experience the consequences. It is true
that women demand a lot from men. It is true and the opposite. Because of this, ladies do respect and appreciate
men who **prove with actions** their commitment to the
mutual betterment.

Do you remember the last time you made a **major commitment** in front of yourself? 4 years ago, I was enjoying
my evening "sahaja yoga meditation" and was watching
a lecture of Dr. Shri Mataji. At one time, she suddenly
made a noticeable pause and looking me right in the eye
from the screen said: "There are so many problems in
this world. You have to decide whether you will be part of
them or part of their solutions!" This was a **very strong
moment** for me, which I still clearly remember. It moved
and provoked something in me. I placed a hand on my
heart and said to myself: "From now one I promise to **be
part of the solutions**!" So far, I stick to my promise and
this book is one of the proofs.

I know first hand that it is never easy to commit yourself
to doing something or ask yourself big questions, which
require tough answers. As you already know, I reached
the point for good or bad to ask myself: "Will I continue
to live?" After I gave a positive answer, I asked myself
a tougher question: "**Why**?" The ability to ask and be
asked tough questions is one of the requirements to **be at
the top** because this is the main job there. Another also
very important ability is to **set clear goals and achieve
them**.

I could have spend my free time for the last several years
watching TV, taking rest and hanging out with friends.
However, I was thoroughly educating myself going far beyond the "required". One day I wrote the title of this book

and challenged myself to write it no matter how difficult it seemed to me at that time.

Women are genetically programmed to search and get attracted by men who stick to their goals and achieve them. Moreover, they adore **determined men**. That's why it is very important to <u>know exactly what you want</u> from a relationship with a girl and **state it clearly**.

Regardless of what a woman sees rationally in you, her unconsciousness will definitely scan you as a **potential father** of her children. If you pass this check, she will be interested in you. Otherwise, she will move to the **next one**. That's why it is extremely important to look and really **be reliable, committed and results-oriented man**. Add to this **win-win thinking** and you will be very attractive in the eyes of most women.

However, you need **only one** out of 3 billion women. Many guys find it difficult to break up with girlfriends, who are **not appropriate any more**. They are afraid to hurt them and themselves. I **never** have such problems because of the following win-win concept.

- I want the very best for you and me. Because of first, second, third, we are **not** a great match. That's why our best option is to break up and continue searching for Mr. and Ms. really Perfect.

If I cannot make her **very happy** but selfishly keep her next to me, I am **not** doing anyone a favour. Breaking a new relationship at the moment when there is a <u>significant difference or problem</u> proves my commitment to the utmost mutual well-being. Women **understand and accept** this concept because it is the best for them as well.

An iron rule when I start a relationship with a woman is to tell her the following. "The moment you aggressively raise your voice you have a **final warning**. If this happens again you are out of my life **irreversibly and forever**!" It works. I do want to get married and several studies prove the positive effects from it.

However, when I give **100% respect, love and care** I will **never** accept to face actions, which will suppress the optimal condition of my body, mind and soul. I have heard that if you really want something you must **be ready to leave without turning back**. I am 24 hours/day, 365 days/year **ready**!

If it is for the sake of having children, we live in an overcrowded world. There are so many children and teenagers. It is enough to look in their big innocent eyes, which beg for some **genuine attention and care**, and frank and serious answers to their questions often posted online. I do my best to be of help for them.

It is your universal and constitutional right to **be respected**! This is **crucial** to be able to develop and flourish physically, mentally and spiritually. It does **not** matter what kind of relationship has a person with you, who unreasonably and consistently **suppresses** and "**suffocates**" you with ill-treatment. You <u>must do something</u> about that. Try with good by talking with them and discussing how their behaviour affects you negatively.

If they keep on suffocating you, **determinately** warn them to **stop doing it**! If this also does **not** solve the problem, consider the following. Any person for whom there is something more important than your well-being and inner confidence, peace and development, is **definitely NOT worth being part of your life!**

No one should stand over your head and always interfere with your decisions, plans and actions. No one has the right to make you doubt in your abilities, talents, confidence and chances for success. That's why think very carefully to whom you allow to be a **vocal** in your life. Personally, I give such status to people who tell me their opinion **only if I ask** them.

What I do with the rest who start pouring advice without even knowing in details a topic. I politely remind them for their **limited knowledge** and that I take into consideration **only experts' opinions**. This immediately shuts their big mouths and shows them that you are **not** Tom, Dick or Harry who can be manipulated as a doll on strings.

If you also **think win-win,** it becomes **impossible** to do something, which will hurt yourself or another person. If you are concerned that after breaking up with a girl you may not find another for a long time, I want to stress again the importance to **stand out**. We live in a world where a handful of "smart" people do their best to **unisex** and **depersonalize** the masses. They tell everyone how to think, how to dress and behave all in one way.

With the aggressive invasion of "unisex" names, clothes, perfumes and products even the differences between the genders start to diminish. As a result, the individual simply **disappears** in a grey unisex ocean.

On the contrary, what make those at the top? **They stand out in every single aspect!** They **never** follow fashion, stereotypes or patterns. Just the opposite. **They create them**. That's why they are at the top and they are **Alpha** or leading the show. The rest who blindly follow them range from Beta to Zeta. Are these national and international famous people and celebrities from Venus or Mars? No, because they eat, sleep and have sex just like you. Then what's the difference? They have realized that you either <u>lead or follow</u> the show. There is **NO middle option**.

Nowadays, when even "experts" are corrupted from affiliations with big companies, which sponsor their research, is crazy to trust **100% anyone**. Personally, I will give **maximum 95% confidence** even to the leading authorities in the world on a certain subject. If I have to make a decision based on their statements, I will <u>double and even triple check them</u> with other independent resources. Then and only then I will be sure that their advice are worth complying.

When it comes to **your** health and future, **never** leave yourself entirely in the hands of **only one** person. The least you can do is to **check their suggestions**. Humans quite often make mistakes. Thousands of people die annually because of physicians' mistakes. I have read cancer survivors stories, which have wowed me. The patients start following the advice from their doctor and because medicine still cannot do anything about advanced stages, they come very close to death.

At certain moment, the patients realize that if **they** do not take their life in their hands, they will die in **a few months**. They search for alternative treatments and when their doctors call them for yet another dose of radiation, they refuse. Then the physicians started shouting on the phone threatening that without it in 2-3 months they would be dead. Well, these people are **still alive after 5-7 years!** They have realized that "<u>I am the Master of my life and destiny</u>!" and have acted accordingly. I hope that you do **not** have to become a "survivor" from a terminal disease to **realize and energize it every single day of your life**.

Sex Business 301: Make Her Emotionally Attached to Your Outstanding Bed

You will spend almost **half of your life sleeping**. It is definitely **not** necessary to be a millionaire to spend this half in **luxury**. In addition, if you are serious about making loyal a **hot lady** then **trash any cheap cotton bed linen**. Probably you have some idea what great everyday efforts women do to maintain their skin in perfect condition. Cotton sheets start to pill in several months, becoming rough and unpleasant on touch. In addition, most of the men out there will offer her an ordinary bed and cotton bed linen. This is an excellent chance for you to **stand out** from the rest. How?

There is one type of material used for the production of underwear to suits, which is **the very best** in each aspect. It is the most

- smooth on touch
- sexy
- luxurious
- durable
- year long appropriate
- versatile
- keeps you cool in the winter
- keeps you warm in the summer
- women are crazy about it

I am sure that every lady out there will agree that there is **nothing better** than to wear and sleep covered in... **silk**. That's why on my bed there is only the girls' favourite bed linen. You may object that silk is "very expensive". I know. In addition, from visual point of view it is **not** very impressive. That's why I will share a combination, which is cheaper and visually incredible. The first component is **sandwashed silk**. This is a specially washed pure silk, which gives it **addictive** smoothness and mesmerizing shining. Compared to non-washed in this way silk, it is <u>significantly more affordable</u>.

The second type is **silk charmeuse**. This is a specially woven material which from one side is pure silk while from the other is synthetic shining satin. This combination makes it very smooth on the silk side, which touches your skin and is incredible shining on the other cover side. When you combine your bed linen from these 2 very special types of silk, the result is **mesmerizing** for the girls. In addition, it is more affordable for the guys.

Here is a trick I use to create a **smashing impression** for the bed. The bottom and top sheet and 2 pillowcases, which touch the skin, are from 100% natural **sandwashed silk**. The **duvet cover** and the pillowcases of 2 additional pillows for decoration are from **silk charmeuse**. Their satin-shining side is on the top.

When a girl looks at my bed, she sees the glittering silk charmeuse set of the duvet cover and the 2 additional pillows. When we go to sleep, I remove the extra pillows. In this way, we sleep covered in the sandwashed silk sheets and pillowcases, which are simply fascinating on touch. In terms of visual effect, smoothness and cost effectiveness, this is **the best combination in the world**.

The silk bed linen comes in 5 main colours. My personal favourite, which stands out from the rest, is "**pearl grey**". This is silver with a hint of blue. The other colours are very pale and unimpressive. If you want to see how mesmerizing this combination is, make a search at <u>www. froogle.com</u>. There you can see pictures next to each result. Here are the best keyword phrases you can use:

silk charmeuse duvet covers pearl grey

sandwashed silk bed sheets pearl grey

With a good quality mattress and such bed linen, every girl that you bring at home will readily jump on your bed. So far, the only problems I have had were getting girls **out of my silky bed**. After all, people quickly get used to such extras. I do believe that if <u>you</u> do **not** pamper yourself, **no one will do it**. Moreover, you will score many extra points with such an <u>outstanding and addictive bed</u>. As the most durable material, anything made from silk can **outlive you**. This is a "once in a lifetime" type of purchase which is really worth it and deserves to be thought out carefully.

Do you Feel Hot and Sexy in Your Underwear

I bet that you love to see your girlfriend or wife wearing **sexy underwear**. Well, the same is true for them. Am I going to praise all those brands of men's underwear, which are aggressively advertised everywhere? Oh, no. Let the guy next door sweat in overpriced Calvin Klein's cotton underwear. You may opt for the more affordable and **really the best money can buy**. Can you guess the material, which provides <u>unbelievable</u> thermal and moisture management year-round and looks so sexy that creates <u>mouth-watering reaction in women</u>? It is of course the…**silk**.

The first time when I put on "men's silk knit boxer briefs" and "men's silk knit leopard tank top" I loved them so much that I trashed **all** my cotton underwear. Since then I have no intentions to go back to it. If you compare the prices, they are very similar. However, the difference for you is **HUGE!**

There is nothing more **common and boring** than white cotton underwear. In addition, it makes you sweat a lot when it is hot. 100% silk men's underwear has exactly the opposite qualities and additional ones. Just try it once and I guarantee you that even if someone offers you free Calvin Klein's underwear, you will **not** take it.

Is silk used only for bed linen and underwear? Not at all and the following keywords will assist you to pinpoint the best in sleepwear, loungewear and casual dressing. Once again, www.froogle.com displays pictures so you can see immediately how something looks. In addition, the option for sorting according to price gives you match-es, which are perfectly affordable for you. The following keyword phrases are divided in 3 categories:

100% Silk Underwear

"silk men's underwear" -satin -charmeuse
"men's silk knit " -satin -charmeuse
"100% silk boxer shorts " -satin -charmeuse
"men's silk knit boxer briefs " -satin -charmeuse
"100% Silk boxer shorts" -satin -charmeuse
"silk twist boxer briefs" -satin -charmeuse
"silk lounge boxer short" -satin -charmeuse
"men's silk knit tank top" -satin -charmeuse

Silk Sleepwear and Loungewear

Classic silk pajama
silk stripe pajama
Silk kimono
Classic silk robe
Silk robe
Silk full-length robe" -satin -charmeuse

"Silk lounge pants" -satin -charmeuse

Silk Shirts and T-shirts

Morelia long sleeve silk t-shirt
Silk knit t-shirt
Banded collar silk shirt
Patterned silk shirt
Squiggle-stripe short sleeve silk shirt

Do you have an Outstanding Grooming 365 Days per Year?

- (the door bell rings and I open the door) Hello. My name is Sandy and I am your new neighbour.
- Oh, that's great. Nice to meet you. Would you like a cup of tea made from the herb, which for centuries has been the secret of the most beautiful women in the Chinese Empire?
- I would love to.
- Please come in.

Now imagine that my hair or home was a **complete mess**. Could I have the confidence in front of this new great girl to sell myself right away and really impress her? **For sure not.** If you are **not** married then Ms. Perfect can pop up in front of you **any time and anywhere**. If you have already made it, then the girl of your dreams is with you every day. In both cases, it is very important to look your best every single day. Why? Because the other guys do **not** pay a lot of attention to their appearance and this is another chance for you to stand out.

I was amazed that my sister spends **minimum 10 minutes** in front of the mirror before going to... throw the trash! For me this was ridiculous. However, gradually I also realized that it does **not** matter whether you are at home or somewhere out. You **have to** look great from tip to toe. After all another Sandy can always knock on your door and if you do **not** grab her attention, she will go to check the guy next door.

That's why I have a challenge for you. Spend **10 minutes** carefully examining your appearance from tip to toe. To grab or to maintain the attention of a lady you have to score high in **her** eyes. Instead of guessing and risking missing something important, I asked each of my girlfriends to participate in the creation of the following **"Smashing (First) Impression Checklist"**.

- Perfect, short and sexy haircut
- Clean and shining hair
- No hairs showing from your nose
- No hairs between your eyebrows
- Perfectly combed and trimmed eyebrows
- Bright and vivid eyes
- No dark circles and deep wrinkles below your eyes
- Clean, youthful and radiant skin on the face
- Perfectly shaved face and trimmed underarms
- Bright and healthy smile
- Clean, pink tongue
- Fresh breathe and moderate quantity of a brand perfume
- Soft, kissable lips
- Take a shower every morning
- Use daily pleasant and mildly scented antiperspirant
- Regularly trim the hair all over your body
- Wear good quality clothes and sexy underwear
- Perfectly clean, trimmed and shining nails
- Smooth hands
- Perfectly shaved testicles and anus

- Anal cleaning (douche) during the morning shower
- Show some flesh (unbutton the top 1-2 buttons or wear sleeveless/short sleeve T-shirt, blouse, etc)
- Wear yellow-gold chain on your neck or a wrist bracelet
- Regularly workout for a lean and ripped body
- Maintain nice tan throughout the year using solarium

I think that these 25 points will assist you to look really your very best in the eyes of every lady out there. A man who follows these guidelines for perfect grooming will definitely stand out from the crowd and look like **a world-class sex service professional**.

Many men complain directly or indirectly that women do **not** pay a lot of attention to them. Also around 50% of all married couples end up with a **divorce**. I am sure that significant part of this group of problems is the decline in men's self-commitment to look and feel at their best **every day**. While they actively date or enjoy honeymoon, men pay great attention to details. **Why should this stop**?

Can you imagine the following honeymoon couple? The lady is reading Daniel Steel in the bed while the guy is watching porn movies. I cannot. Why they should passively lie next to each other and only **dream** about romanticism, passion and sex? If you want your life to be a **non-stop honeymoon** then stick non-stop to the checklist. In addition, consciously do your male's duty as if you are a **world class sex professional.** Then your lady will never think about other guy, Daniel Steel and soap operas.

Advanced Sex Business: Satisfaction and Loyalty Defined in the Philosophy of #1 Luxury Hotel Chain in the World

Have you heard of **The Ritz-Carlton**® Luxury Hotel Chain? The secret for their incredible success and non-stop growth is their **unique philosophy**. It has emerged as a necessity and key to success throughout the decades. A very small percentage of all hotel guests can afford to stay at their hotels. That's why they also do **whatever it takes** to make their guests <u>totally satisfied and loyal</u> as the only way to tell them in the future: "Welcome back."

They definitely know how to **stand out** from the several other 5-star hotel chains and do succeed to make most of their guests **loyal**. That's why I have followed their example creating a two-part philosophy for achieving and maintaining **the ultimate relationship** with a girl.

The Relationship Credo

Our home is a place
where the **genuine** care
and comfort of each other is
our highest mission.

I pledge to provide the finest
personal attention and service
to my partner, who will always
enjoy a romantic, passionate, yet
relaxed ambience.

The experience of living
together instills well-being
and fulfills even the **unexpressed**

wishes and needs of each other.

The Mutual Promise

we nurture the
relationship to the benefit of
each other and the couple
by applying the principles of trust,
honesty, respect and loyalty.

We foster a home environment
where quality of life is enhanced,
individual aspirations are fulfilled
and the mutual sense of bliss is
strengthened.

It is true that in certain aspects, I am very tough with women and I should be. That's why I never think twice to energize the adapted Ritz-Carlton Basic 16: **Escort the girl to the front door**. At the same time each one of my girlfriends has received "the finest personal service" and has felt just like a princess at my home.

This **controversial approach** maintains some mystic and unpredictability, which definitely **fascinates women**. An Alpha Male has to repetitively challenge himself. Moreover, his only concern should be how to **stand out** from the crowd of guys in the bed, at home, on the street, at work and <u>everywhere</u>.

I often ask myself: What does the crowd of men do… about sex? They watch many porn movies. What will I do to stand out? I will write a bestseller on multiple orgasms. Will I **score many extra points** in the eyes of **great girls** if I achieve it? Oh, yes. Then let's do it. What the crowd of men do… after work? They splash in front of the TV and eat junk food. What will I do to stand out? In the evening, I eat mostly vegetables and fruits plus walking or doing fitness. If you really want to stand out from the rest, you can find **100s of ways to do it!** The same is true for achieving great success in life.

History gives us many examples of men who have started from the **zero** and have made it to the world's top. Take for example **Rockefeller**. As a small boy, he started to sell apples and gradually became a **household name** for a rich and successful man. Take as another example **Caesar Ritz**. He has started as an ordinary waiter and gradually has become the "Hotelier of Kings and King of Hoteliers". If they and many others have done it, **everyone can do it**.

The ultimate goal of this book is to educate and empower you to make the steps towards the **ultimate** in your sexual abilities, health and potency. However, there are related macro aspects in life. There if you also want to achieve something significant you have to **be tough** and **know exactly what you want.** I am confident that with the knowledge from this book you will achieve very significant results in a crucial area- **your sexuality**.

Then already having a strong foundation I do expect from you to continue on your way to The Top! Many people have made it and many will make it. **Be one of them** and then I am sure that you will enjoy a fantastic personal and sexual life! Set it as a **goal**, outline an **action plan** and **start working on it from today!**

Conclusion

I deeply believe that this increasingly complicated world needs more high-testosterone men who have plenty of confidence, courage and sense of responsibility. Only such men determinately take up their sleeves and do their best to solve a myriad of challenges.

"Men who for truth and honor's sake
Stand fast and suffer long.
Brave men who work while others sleep,
Who dare while others fly...
They build a nation's pillars deep
And lift them to the sky." by Ralph Waldo Emerson

I am thankful to the Divine for giving me the mind, patience and persistence to study in great details the incredibly complex human biochemistry and metabolism. I am also thankful for my commitment to excellence and the betterment of the world. Thank you for giving me the opportunity to be of assistance for your betterment and further development. I would like to finish the book with the following outstanding quote:

"**I will act now.** I will act now. I will act now. Henceforth, I will repeat these words each hour, each day, everyday, until the words become as much a **habit** as my breathing, and the **action, which follows,** becomes as instinctive as the blinking of my eyelids. With these words, I can condition my mind to perform every action necessary for **my success. I will act now.** I will repeat these words repeatedly and again.

I will walk where failures fear to walk. I will work when failures seek rest. I will act now for **now is all I have**. Tomorrow is the day reserved for the labor of the lazy. I am **not** lazy. Tomorrow is the day when the failure will succeed. I am **not** a failure. I will act **now**. Success will **not** wait. If I delay, success will become wed to another and lost to me forever. **This is the time. This is the place. I am the person.**" by Og Mandino

Bibliographical References

I hope that in the future you will be motivated enough by the book to look at different journals researches and studies because they often provide **invaluable** information for achieving the ultimate.

References for L-Arginine

1. Wolf A; Zalpour C; Theilmeier G; et al; Dietary L-Arginine Supplementation Normalizes Platelet Aggregation in Hypercholesterolemia Humans. J Am. Coll. Cardiol; 1997; 29: 479-85.
2. Reyes AA; Karl E, Klahr S., Role of Arginine in Health and in Renal Disease. Am. J. Phuysiol; 1994; 267: F-331-F-346. Besset, A., Bonardet A., Ron Douin G; et al. Increase in sleep related GH and PRL secretion after chronic Arginine Aspartate administration in Man. ACTA Endocrinal 1982; 99: 18-23.
3. Alternative Medical Review. 2002, Dec;7 (6):512-22.
4. Appleton, J. 2002. Arginine: Clinical potential of a semi-essential amino.
5. Pryor J.P., Blandy J.P., Evans P et al, Controlled Clinical Trial of Arginine for Infertile Men with Oligospermia. BR. J UROL. 1978; 50; 47-50.

6. Nakaki T; Kato R. 1994. Beneficial circulatory effect of L-arginine. Japanese Journal of Pharmacology. Oct, 66:2, 167-71
7. Reyes AA; Karl IE; Klahr S Role of arginine in health and in renal disease (editorial) American Journal of Physiology, 1994 Sep, 267:3 Pt 2, F331-46
8. Albina JE, Mills CD, Barbul A, Thirkill CE, Henry WL Jr, Mastrofrancesco B, Caldwell MD. Arginine metabolism in wounds. American Journal of Physiology 1988;254:E459-E467.
9. Bode-Boger SM; Boger RH, Kienres., Junrer W., Frolich JC, Elevated L-Arginine/Dimethylarginine Ration Contributes to Enhanced Systemic NO Production by Dietary L-Arginine in Hypercholesterolemic Rabbits, Biochem. Biophys. Res. Commun. 1996; 20 (12 Suppl) 5:60-562.

References for Choline

1. Groff, J and Gropper, S. Advanced Nutrition and Human Metabolism. 541-543, 2000.
2. Conlay L, et al. Int J Sports Med. 13 Suppl 1:S141-2, 1992.

References for L-Tyrosine

1. Banderet, LE, and Lieberman HR. Treatment with tyrosine, a neurotransmitter precursor, reduces environmental stress in humans. Brain Res Bull 22: 759-762, 1989.
2. Gelenberg AJ, Gibson CJ, Wojcik JD. Neurotransmitter precursors for the treatment of depression. Psychopharmacol Bull 1982;18:7-18.
3. Meyer JS, Welch KMA, Deshmuckh VD, et al. Neurotransmitter precursor amino acids in the treat-

ment of multi-infarct dementia and Alzheimer's disease. J Am Geriatr Soc 1977;7:289-98.

4. Lieberman, HR, Corkin S, Spring BJ, Wurtman RJ, and Growden JH. The effects of dietary neurotransmitter precursors on human behavior. Am J Clin Nutr 42: 366-370, 1985.

5. Wurtman, RJ, and Lewis MC. Exercise, plasma composition and neurotransmission. In: Advances in Nutrition and Top Sport, edited by Brouns F.. Basel: Karger, 1991, vol. 32, p. 94-109.

6. Romanowski, W, and Grabiec S. The role of serotonin in the mechanism of central fatigue. Acta Physiol Pol 25: 127-134, 1974.

References for 5-HTP

1. Angst J, Woggon B, Schoepf J 1977 Oct "The treatment of depression with L-5-hydroxytryptophan versus imipramine. Results of two open and one double-blind study." Arch Psychiatr Nervenkr. 224(2), 175-86

2. Meyers S 2000 Feb "Use of neurotransmitter precursors for treatment of depression.". Altern Med Rev 5(1), 64-71

3. den Boer JA, Westenberg HG 1990 Mar "Behavioral, neuroendocrine, and biochemical effects of 5-hydroxytryptophan administration in panic disorder." Psychiatry Res 31(3), 267-78

References for cGMP, NO, PGE-1, PDE-5 and Icariin

1. TF Lue, KL Lee. Pharmacotherapy for erectile dysfunction. Chin Med J (Engl), 2000; 113: 291-8.

2. Knispel HH, Goessl C, Beckman R. Nitric oxide mediates relaxation in rabbit and human corpus cavernosum smooth muscle. Urol Res 1992; 20: 253-7.
3. Buvat J, Lemaire A, Herbaut-Buvat M. Intracavernosal pharmacotherapy: comparison of moxisylyte and prostaglandin E1. J Impt Res 1996; 8: 41-6.
4. Otani T. Intracavernous injection test by prostaglandin E1. Nippon Rinsho 2002; 60 (Suppl 6): 173-7.
5. Lue T F. Erectile Dysfunction. N Engl J Med 2000; 342: 1802-13.
6. Burnett AL, Lowenstein CJ, Bredt DS, Chang TSK, Snyder SH. Nitric oxide: a physiologic mediator of penile erection. Science 1992; 257: 401-3.
7. Lin CS, Ho HC, Chen KC, Lin G, Nunes L, Lue TF. Intra-cavernosal injection of vascular endothelial growth factor induces nitric oxide synthase isoform. BJU Int 2002; 89: 955-60.
8. Pietta PG, Mauri PL, Manera E, Ceva PL, Rava A. An approved HPLC determination of flavonoids in medical plant extracts. Chromatographia 1989; 27: 509-12.
9. Xin ZC. Kim EK, Tian ZJ, Lin GT, Guo YL. Icariin on relaxation of corpus cavernosm smooth muscle. Chin Sci Bulle 2001; 46: 485-9.
10. Qiao L, Xin ZC, Fu J, Liu WJ, Lin GT, Chen S. Expression of Phosphodiesterase 5 in clitoris cavernosum and effect of Icariin on cGMP levels in vitro. Chin J Urol 2002; 23: 670-2.
11. Fu J, Qiao L, Jin TY, Lin GT, Wang YY, Xin ZC. Effects of Icariin on cGMP synthesis in corpus cavernosm of rabbits. Chinese Phamarcological Bulletin 2002; 18: 430-2.
12. Liang HR, Vuorela P, Vuorela H, Hiltinen R. Isolation and immunomodulatory effect of flavonol glycosides from epimedium hunense. Plants Med 1997; 63: 316-9.

13. Du Q, Xia M, Ito Y. Purification of icariin from the extract of Epimedium segittatum using high-speed counter-current chromatography. J Chromatogr A 2002; 962: 239-41.
14. Linuma M, tanaka T, Sakakibara N, Mizuno M, Matsuda H, Shiomoto H, et al. Phagocytic activity of leaves of epimedium species on mouse reticuloen-dothelial system. Yakugaku Zasshi 1990; 110: 179-85.
15. Lee MK, Choi YJ, Sung SH, Shin DI, Kim JW, Kim YC. Antihepatotoxic activity of icariin, a major con-stituent of epimedium koreanum. Planta Med 1995; 61: 523-6.
16. He W, Sun H, Yang B, Zhang D, Kabelitz D. Immunoregulatory effects of the herba epimediia gly-coside icariin. Arzneimittel-forschung 1995; 45: 910-3.
17. Zheng J, Luo Y, Meng X, Sun Y, Zhang Y, Dong X, et al. Effects of Sichuan herba epimedii on the con-centration of plasma middle molecular substances and sulfhydryl group of "Yang-deficiency" model ani-mal. Chung Kuo Chung Yao Tsa Chih 1995; 20: 238-9.
18. Boolell M, Allen MJ, Ballard SA, Gepi-Attes S, Muirhead GJ, Naylor AM, et al. Sildenafil:a orally ac-tive type 5 cyclic GMP-specific phosphodiesterase inhibitor for the treatment of penile erectile dysfunc-tion. Int J Impot Res 1996; 8: 47-52.
19. Francis SH, Turko IV, Corbin JD. Cyclic nucleotide phospho-diesterases: relating structure and function. Prog Nucleic Acid Res Mol Biol 2001; 65: 1-52.
20. Soderling SH, Beavo JA. Regulation of cAMP and cGMP signaling: new phosphodiesterases and new functions. Curr Opin Cell Biol 2000; 12: 174-9.
21. Loughney K and Ferguson K. Identification and quantification of PDE isozymes and subtypes by molecular biological methods. In: Schudt C, Dent G,

Rabe KF, editors. Phosphodiesterase inhibitors. San Diego: Academic Press; 1996. 99: 1-19.
22.Lin CS, Chow S, Lau A, Tu R, Lue. Human PDE5A gene encodes three PDE5 isoforms from two alternate phospho-diesterases: functional implications of multiple isoforms. Phyiol Rev 1995; 75: 725-8.

References for Prostate

1. Merck Manual, 14th ed., pp 1566-1567
2. Fair and Heston, 1977; Pfeiffer, 1978
3. Taylor, D. S. "Nutrients Can Remedy Prostate Problems," Today's Living, February 1990, pp 12-13
4. Wall Street Journal, April 22, 1992
5. Soybean Products May Lower Prostate Cancer," Lancaster Intelligencer-Journal, January 12, 1994
6. Prostate Cancer Cure Questioned, The Associated Press, January 27, 1994
7. USA Weekend, December 3-5, 1993, p 14)
8. Balch and Balch, Prescription for Nutritional Healing, Avery Publishing, Garden City Park, NY, 1990, pp 271-273
9. Fair, W. R. and Heston, W. "Prostate Inflammation Linked to Zinc Shortage" Prevention 113: June, 1977
10.Hennenfent BR. The economics of urological care in the 21st century [letter]. Urology 1996;47:285-6.
11. Weidner W, Schiefer HG, Krauss H, Jantos CH, Freidrich HJ, Altmannsberger M. "Chronic prostatitis" a thorough search for etilogically involved microorganisms in 1,461 patients. Infection 1991;19:S119-25.
12.Krieger JN, Egan KJ, Ross SO, Jacobs R, Berger RE. Chronic pelvic pains represent the most prominent urogenital symptoms of "chronic prostatitis." Urology 1996;48:715-22.

13. Stamey TA. Pathogenesis and treatment of urinary tract infections. Baltimore: Williams and Wilkins, 1980.
14. McNeal J. Regional morphology and pathology of the prostate. Am J Clin Pathol 1968;49:347-57.
15. Bostrom K. Chronic inflammation of the male accessory sex glands and its affect on the morphology of the spermatozoa. Scand J Urol Nephrol 1971;5:133.
16. Kohnen PW, Drach GW. Patterns of inflammation in prostatic hyperplasia: a histologic and bacteriologic study. J Urol 1979;121:755-60.
17. Gerson, Max A Cancer Therapy: Results of 50 Cases, Gerson Institute, P.O. Box 430, Bonita, CA 91908
18. Pfeiffer, C. Zinc and Other Micro-nutrients, Keats, 1978 pp 46-47

References for Testosterone

1. Seeley, R.R., T.D. Stephens and P. Tate (1998). Anatomy and Physiology (4th edition). WCB McGraw-Hill.
2. Arnold, A.M. et al. Journal of Endocrinology. 150, 291-399, 1996.
3. Beato, M. Cell. 56, 335-344, 1989.
4. Norman, A.W. and G. Litwack (1987). Hormones. Academic Press, Inc.
5. Berg, J. Cell. 57, 1065-1068, 1989.
6. Braunstien, G.D. in Basic and Clinical Endocrinology, Greenspan F.S. and Strewler G.J. eds. Appleton and Lange, Stanford CT, 403-433, 1997.
7. Bullock, L.P. et al. Endocrinology. 94, 746-748, 1974.
8. Casaburi, R., T. Storer and S. Bhasin (1996). Androgen Effects on Body Composition and Muscle Performance. In: Pharmacology, Biology, and

Clinical Applications of Androgens (Bhasin et al. Eds), Wiley-Liss.

9. Hurel SJ, et al. Relationship of physical exercise and ageing to growth hormone production. Clin Endocrinol (Oxf) 1999 Dec;51(6):687-91.

10. Chang, C. et al. Proc Natl Acad Sci USA, 85: 7211-7215, 1988.

11. Christiansen, K. in Testosterone Action, Deficiency, and Substitution, Nieschlag, E. and Behre, H.M. eds. Springer-Verlag, New York, 107-142, 1998.

12. Culig, Z. et al. World J Urol. 13, 285-289, 1995.

13. Dahlberg, E. et al. Endocrinol. 108, 1431-36, 1981.

14. Colker, C.M., J. Antonio and D. Kalman. The metabolism of orally ingested 19-nor-4-androstene-3, 17-dione and 19-nor-4-androstene-3, 17-diol in healthy, resistance-trained man. Journal of Strength and Conditioning Research, 15(1): 144-147, 2001.

15. Marks, D.B., A.D. Marks and C. Smith (1996). Basic Medical Biochemistry. Williams and Wilkins.

16. Danhaive, P.A. and Rousseau, G.G. J Steroid Biochem Mol Biol. 24, 481-487, 1986.

17. Danhaive, P.A. and Rousseau, G.G. J Steroid Biochem Mol Biol. 29, 575-581, 1988.

18. Evans, R.M. Science. 240, 889-893, 1988.

19. Fang, Y. et al. J Biol Chem. 271 (45), 28697-28702, 1996.

20. Freedman, L.P. Endocr Rev. 13, 129-145, 1992.

21. Gouras GK, et al. Testosterone reduces neuronal secretion of Alzheimer's beta-amyloid peptides. Proc Natl Acad Sci U S A 2000 Feb 1;97(3):1202-5

22. Guyton, A.C. (1991). Textbook of Medical Physiology (8th edition). W.B. Saunders

23. Gloyna, R.E. and Wilson, J.D. J Clin Endocrinol. 29, 970-973, 1969.

24. Grino, P.B. et al. Endocrinol. 120, 1914-1920, 1987.

25. Saartok, T. Int J Sports Med. 5, 130-136, 1984.

26. Hsiao, P.W. J Biol Chem. 32, 22373-22379, 1999.

27. Laio, S. et al. J Steroid Biochem. 34, 41-51, 1989.
28. Jenster, G. et al. Biochem J. 293, 761-768, 1993.
29. Peterziel, H. et al. In Verhoeven, G., and Swinnen, J.V. Molecular and Cellular Endocrinology. 151, 205-212, 1999.
30. Hickson, R.C. et al. Med Sci Sports Exerc. 22, 331-340, 1990.
31. Gustafsson, J. et al. In Hormones and Cancer, Gurpide, E. et al. eds. Alan R. Liss, Inc. New York, 261-290, 1984.
32. Kadi, F. et al. Histochem Cell Biol. 113, 25-29, 2000.
33. Yeh, S. et al. Proc Natl Acad Sci USA. 93 (11), 5517-5521, 1996.

Printed in the United States
63984LVS00004B/1-39